Spontaneous
Happiness

Spontaneous Happiness

A New Path to Emotional Well-Being

Andrew Weil, MD

LITTLE, BROWN AND COMPANY
New York Boston London

Little, Brown and Company
Hachette Book Group
1290 Avenue of the Americas, New York, NY 10104
littlebrown.com

Originally published in hardcover by Little, Brown and Company, November 2011.

First paperback edition, January 2013.

Little, Brown and Company is a division of Hachette Book Group. The Little, Brown name and logo are trademarks of Hachette Book Group, Inc.

Library of Congress Cataloging-in-Publication Data

Weil, Andrew.
    Spontaneous happiness / Andrew Weil. — 1st ed.
        p. cm.
    Includes bibliographical references and index.
    ISBN 978-0-316-12944-2 (hc) / 978-0-316-12942-8 (pb)
    1. Mental health.   2. Mind and body.   3. Emotions.   4. Happiness.   5. Well-being.
I. Title.
    RA790.W45 2011
    613—dc23   2011020096

10 9 8 7 6 5 4 3

LSC-C

Printed in the United States of America

Contents

Spontaneous Happiness

Introduction

I n the early 1970s, I lived in Colombia, studying native uses of medicinal and psychoactive plants. During my stay I made a number of trips to the Vaupés Department of the Amazon basin to visit a tribe of Cubeo Indians. To get there, I had to drive from the capital city of Bogotá at eight thousand feet above sea level to a city in the lower, warmer eastern plains, then take a cargo plane to the tiny frontier town of Mitú in the rain forest. From there it was a half-day trip by motorboat to the Cubeo village. The climate was unrelievedly hot and steamy, and once in the village, I had a very limited range of foods and drinks. When I was not interviewing Cubeos or accompanying them on walks through the rain forest, I spent hours in a hammock under a mosquito net, mostly dreaming about ice-cold drinks.

In particular, I could not stop thinking about my favorite juice bar on Seventh Avenue in downtown Bogotá and the delicious, icy drinks it offered, made from combinations of fresh fruit both familiar and exotic. One that I found irresistible whenever I was in the vicinity was *jugo de maracuyá*, made from a kind of passion fruit, with just enough sugar to offset its natural tartness and just the right amount of crushed ice. I would have given anything to have one as I lay parched and sweating in my hammock in the jungle with nothing to drink but tepid boiled water or tea or the thick, sour beerlike drink *(chicha),* also tepid, that the Indians made from a starchy tuber. If only, I imagined, I could have that cold juice right then and there, I would be supremely happy.

When it came time to leave the Cubeo village, I became obsessed with planning my visit to the juice bar. I pictured myself taking a taxi directly there as soon as I got to Bogotá, but what would I have first? Should I go right for the passion fruit drink of my dreams, or should I build my anticipation and pleasure by starting off with a fresh mango frost? Or maybe a pineapple-coconut shake? Throughout my entire journey—on the boat ride downriver, during what seemed like an endless night in a Mitú flophouse, on the cargo plane (missing its door), and on the long ride to Bogotá—all I could do was contemplate the happiness that was in store for me. But as the road began to climb the eastern foothills of the Andes toward the high plateau of the capital, I felt my anticipation wane as reality intruded on my fantasies. It got cooler and cooler as my trip progressed, and by the time I reached the outskirts of Bogotá, I was in the chill, damp fog that often envelops it. When I was in the jungle and couldn't get it, I had wanted my ice-cold drink. Now that I was close to getting it, I was no longer hot and thirsty and didn't want it nearly as much. By the time I arrived, I was more interested in checking into a hotel and changing into warm clothes than in going to the juice bar. And as I felt the possibility of satisfaction evaporate, my disappointment was compounded by seeing the folly of my fantasies and my tendency to allow myself to be happy on condition of getting something not available in the here and now.

The Harvard psychologist Daniel Gilbert has spent more than a decade studying just how abysmal human beings are at predicting which future events will make them happy. He has found that we tend to overlook how the future context—in my case the climate change I encountered—devalues the happiness potential of the goal we seek, such as the refreshing *jugo.* Here, science confirms the advice of saints and sages over eons: emotional well-being must come from within, because reaching external goals often disappoints.

Clearly, many people today are unhappy. I hear the words "I'm depressed" very often—from patients, friends, colleagues, acquaintances, and strangers—and I've uttered them myself on more than one occasion. But what do people mean when they say they're depressed?

For some, it's nothing more than a way of describing a bad day or being bummed about the weather or about a favorite sports team's loss. Others are admitting they suffer from a chronic mental illness that can be incapacitating. In between is a broad spectrum of negative moods and emotional states, including sadness, pessimism, and the inability to experience pleasure or maintain interest in the potentially joyous and rewarding aspects of life.

The root meaning of the verb *depress* is to "push down." To be depressed is to have one's mood or spirits lowered. Who or what does the pushing? And how can we define *down* except as relative to something else? What is the emotional equivalent of sea level, from which point all positions above or below can be measured? Are we better off hovering near that level, or should we strive to stay above it?

These questions interest me greatly, in my ongoing efforts to both come to terms with the changing contours of my own emotions and understand why so many people today are experiencing depression. Also, I'm not sure how to respond to the question "Are you happy?," which I get asked frequently. *Happy* might mean "content," "joyful," "blissed out," or simply not sad. And how happy am I—or is anyone—supposed to be? There are self-assessment tools designed to help individuals determine their level of happiness, but I find it frustrating to answer the questions and don't find them useful.*

There are a great many books offering ways to attain happiness, and no shortage of books about depression and its treatment (with or without popular drugs like Prozac). This book is different. It is about

---

* The best is the Oxford Happiness Questionnaire. See http://www.meaningandhappiness .com/oxford-happiness-questionnaire/214/.

emotional well-being, and it is informed by the new science of integrative mental health, a field I helped develop.

Integrative mental health works from the general philosophy of integrative medicine (IM), beginning with an emphasis on the human organism's innate capacity for self-regulation and healing. IM views mind and body as inseparable: two poles of one human being. It takes into account all aspects of lifestyle that influence health and risks of disease. It also makes use of all available methods to maintain health and support healing—both conventional therapies and alternative ones for which there is scientific evidence of efficacy.

I understand *health* as a dynamic condition of wholeness and balance that allows us to move through life and not succumb to malfunctions of our own physiology or suffer harm from all the potentially damaging influences we encounter. If you are healthy, you can interact with germs and not get infections, with allergens and not have allergic reactions, with toxins and not be harmed. Moreover, a healthy person has a reserve of energy that allows for fulfilling engagement with life. The essential qualities of health are resilience and energy.

When I describe health as dynamic, I mean that it is always changing, allowing the organism to find new configurations of balance as external and internal conditions change. Physiologists use the term *homeostasis* to designate this dynamic self-regulation of living organisms. Thanks to it, our bodies are able to maintain relatively constant temperature, blood sugar, tissue chemistry, and so on, despite great variations in environmental conditions and demands. If, as I believe, mind and body are most usefully viewed as two aspects of the one reality of our being, then homeostasis must also be essential to optimum emotional health. By drawing analogies from the science of physiology and by using the principles of integrative medicine, I will try to answer the questions I raised earlier in this introduction.

Let me start by pointing to some new findings about the function of the human heart. Throughout history, and in many diverse cultures, people have regarded the heart as the seat of emotions. Our language reflects this association *(heartwarming, heartbroken, heartaches,* and *heartthrobs);* in written Chinese and Japanese, the same character denotes both heart and mind.* We often feel strong emotions in our chests, probably because continual hormonal and nervous communication between the heart and brain links the activity of these organs.

When I learned to perform physical examinations in medical school, I was taught to first measure a patient's heart rate by timing the pulse in the radial artery at the wrist. I was taught also to determine whether the rate was regular or irregular, and if irregular, whether it was "regularly irregular" (as from benign premature contractions) or "irregularly irregular" (as in atrial fibrillation, a more serious disorder). Most of the patients I examined had regular pulses in the normal range of 70 to 80 beats per minute. I came to regard the healthy heart as a sort of living metronome, ticking away at perfectly regular intervals, and understood that if a heart beat too fast or too slowly or abandoned its regular rhythm, it was not in good shape and could jeopardize general health.

That was back in the late 1960s. Since then, much closer analysis of electrocardiograms has revealed a surprising fact: healthy hearts do not tick like mechanical clocks or metronomes. Rather, the intervals between beats vary slightly in length, and what is more, this heart-rate variability is a fundamental characteristic of cardiac health. Cardiologists now know that loss of heart-rate variability is an early sign of disease; when profound, it is a poor prognostic sign for recovery from a heart attack. We have also discovered ways to maintain and increase heart-rate variability in healthy individuals using combinations of exercise, stress reduction, and mind/body interventions.

You might wonder why the healthy heart beats at varying intervals. I see it as a sign of resilience and flexibility in responding to moment-to-moment changes in the rest of the body. Clearly, extremes of heart rate are abnormal and unhealthy. But *normal* and *healthy* do not mean "static." In this core function of the human body, we can see

---

* Chinese *xin,* Japanese *shin* or *kokoro.*

the reality and importance of dynamic change that is characteristic of health.

Human emotional states also vary, from extremely negative to extremely positive. At one end is total despondency, with the pain of daily experience so unbearable that suicide appears to be the only option. At the other is ecstatic bliss so intense that attending to basic bodily needs is impossible. Examples of the despondent abound; you may very well know such unfortunate people. Examples of those who experience ecstatic bliss are not common today, but I have studied historical accounts of some, such as Ramakrishna Paramahansa (1836–1886), a famous Indian saint. He spent much of his life in a state of "God-intoxication," wandering, dancing, and singing in ecstasy,* while totally neglecting his body. Ordinary people thought him insane, and he would not have survived if his followers had not cared for him.

I'm sure we can agree that such extremes of negative and positive moods are neither normal nor desirable if they persist, but might they — by marking the limits of emotional variation — help us discover the neutral midpoint of emotional health?

I will tell you at the start that I do not consider happiness to be that midpoint. Nor do I regard it as a mood that we should be in all or most of the time. I wrote earlier that I'm not sure what it means to be happy, especially when I consider the root meaning of that word. It derives from *happ*, an Old Norse root meaning "chance" or "luck," and is closely related to the words *happenstance* and *happening*. Clearly, our forebears regarded good fortune as the basis of happiness, putting the source of this much-sought-after emotion out of our control and in the realm of circumstance — not, I would argue, a good placement. Happiness that comes from winning a bet or from another stroke of good luck is temporary and does not change the set point of our emotional

---

* The word *ecstasy* is of Greek origin, meaning "standing outside" — i.e., the soul (or consciousness) is displaced from the body.

variability. Besides, as we all discover, fortune is fickle. If we hitch our moods to it, we are signing up for lows as powerful as any highs.

Nonetheless, I observe that many people seek happiness "out there." They imagine it will come to them if they get a raise, a new car, a new lover, a refreshing glass of juice, or something else they want but do not have. My own experience, repeated many times, is that the actual emotional reward of getting and having is usually much less than the one imagined. All of the recommendations in this book will help you create an internal state of well-being that is relatively impervious to life's transient ups and downs and independent of what you have or don't have.

I said above that I do not consider happiness to be our baseline or most normal mood. Before you accuse me of deceiving you into reading this book by means of a seductive title, let me explain my choice of the word *spontaneous*. I used that same word in the title of a previous book, *Spontaneous Healing*, intended to build confidence in the human body's innate abilities to maintain and repair, regenerate, and adapt to injury and loss. I call these processes spontaneous to indicate that they are natural and that they arise from internal causes, independent of external agencies. This is an important biological fact, one commonly misunderstood and unappreciated by both medical practitioners and patients. The concept of self-healing is a foundational principle of integrative medicine and has long been a focus of my work. I am certain that if people trusted more in the body's potential for self-healing, and if more doctors honored the healing power of nature, there would be much less need for costly health care services and interventions.

The reality of spontaneous healing does not excuse you from doing everything you can to support it with wise lifestyle choices. Nor does it mean that prudent medical care is unnecessary. The term simply calls attention to the fact that healing is an innate capacity of the organism, rooted in nature. By linking the words *spontaneous* and *happiness* I am asking you to question the prevalent habit of making positive emotions dependent on external agencies and to think of happiness as one of many moods available to us if we allow for healthy variability of our emotional life.

My personal opinion is that the neutral position on the mood spectrum—what I called emotional sea level—is not happiness but rather contentment and the calm acceptance that is the goal of many kinds of spiritual practice. From this perspective, it is possible to accept life in its totality, both the good and the bad, and know that everything is all right, just as it should be, including you and your place in the world. Surprisingly, this acceptance does not breed passivity. I have found that I am most effective at creating positive change when I am in this state; energy normally employed to ward off frustration at opposition or fear of failure is instead channeled precisely where it needs to go. Based on the moments I've been able to be there, I am sure that's where I want to be more of the time.

Here are some basic tenets that inform my writing about emotional well-being:

- It is normal and healthy to experience a variable range of moods and emotions both positive and negative.
- Too many people today are being diagnosed with or are experiencing depression.
- It may be normal, healthy, and even productive to experience mild to moderate depression from time to time as part of the variable emotional spectrum, but it is not normal or healthy to get stuck in that mode or to suffer major depression.
- The set point of emotional variability in our society has become displaced too far into the negative zone. Too many of us are sad and discontented.
- It is unrealistic to want to be happy all the time.
- Happiness arises spontaneously from sources within us. Seeking it outside ourselves is counterproductive.
- It is desirable to cultivate contentment and calm serenity as the neutral midpoint of emotional variability.
- It is desirable and important to develop greater flexibility of emotional responsiveness to both the positive and negative aspects of life and the world.

- It is possible to increase emotional resilience and shift one's emotional set point in the direction of greater positivity.
- It is possible to prevent and manage the commonest forms of depression using the comprehensive approach of integrative mental health.
- Achieving optimum emotional well-being is as important as maintaining optimum physical health.

These tenets are not merely my opinions; each is bolstered by a growing body of rigorous scientific research. If you are comfortable with them, I invite you to read further.

In the first chapter of this book I give you a sense of what emotional well-being means, the goal of your journey, and the role that happiness plays in it.

Chapter 2 is an overview of depression, including my understanding of the causes of the current epidemic of it.

Chapter 3 examines the limitations of the biomedical model now dominant in psychiatry, in particular how it has failed to help us prevent depression, treat it effectively in our population, or improve overall emotional wellness. I also share my excitement about the emerging field of integrative mental health and explain how its view of the causes of depression differs from that of the biomedical model.

Chapter 4 presents evidence for the effectiveness of integrating strategies from Eastern and Western psychology to optimize emotional well-being, drawing on both ancient tradition and contemporary neuroscience.

In the second part of this book I provide specific recommendations.

Chapter 5 presents a comprehensive list of body-oriented therapies aimed at supporting emotional wellness.

Chapter 6 focuses on ways of retraining and caring for the mind in order to change mental habits that undermine emotional resilience and keep us stuck in negative moods.

Chapter 7 concerns the importance of attending to the nonphysical dimension of our experience—what I call secular spirituality—in working toward optimum emotional wellness.

A final chapter gives you a detailed guide to help you use these strategies in order to meet your individual needs. Whether you are prone to depression or not, my suggestions will help you develop greater emotional positivity and resilience and contribute to your general health and wellness.

I have made an effort to present the scientific evidence for my recommendations in terms that nonscientists will understand. Readers who would like more information or details about the science of human emotions will find key references to the medical literature in the notes, beginning on page 239. An appendix on page 231 will direct you to sources of further information, products, and services to support you on your journey to optimum emotional well-being.

I will end this introduction with some personal reassurance. Whether you or someone you love is struggling with depression, or whether you just want greater happiness in your life or simply to feel better in difficult and troubling times, I know that the suggestions in these pages will help you. They are all based on sound science and on my own forty years of clinical experience. Take your time with them and put them into practice at your own pace. You *can* feel better—much better—than you do now. I look forward to guiding you on your journey.

PART ONE

===

THEORY

1

What Is Emotional Well-Being?

I do not claim to have attained optimum emotional well-being. Actually, I think that may be a lifetime goal. For me it's an ongoing process that requires awareness, knowledge, and practice. I do know what good emotional health feels like, and that motivates me to keep at the practice. I'd like to share some of my experiences with you.

On occasion, both when things are going well and when they aren't, I have a profound sense that everything is just as it should be, that my opinions about my situation are irrelevant. That realization is freeing. It helps me to stay comfortably in the vicinity of emotional sea level, the zone of contentment and serenity that I mentioned in the introduction.

Let me tell you about two such occasions.

In June 1959, for several weeks before and after my graduation from my public high school in Philadelphia, I was spontaneously happy, not in the usual sense of that word but more from a deep knowing that I was all right, on the right track, doing what I had been put here for. Things were going very well for me that spring. I had great friends, was enjoying good relations with my parents, had the affection and support of excellent teachers, felt ready and excited to leave home, and saw many opportunities opening up before me for travel, adventure, learning, and discovery. I liked myself. I had much to be happy about in the usual sense, much good fortune, but the deeper feeling came from knowing that I was the person I was supposed to be, uniquely equipped to navigate the world and meet any challenges I might confront. I thought I would be able to maintain that feeling always. It did stay with me for many days and it does return. Whenever it comes back, I am grateful.

Forty-seven years later, at the end of July 2006, I was awakened by an unusually early phone call at my summer retreat in British Columbia. My medical associate Dr. Brian Becker told me that a flash flood had devastated my property in the desert outside Tucson. My first question was "Is anyone hurt?" I was much relieved to hear that the two people staying there had escaped unharmed when a fourteen-foot wall of water came through the property in the middle of the night. My office building had taken the worst hit. Over the next few hours and days, I learned that all of my files, most of my personal papers, and many of my books were lost. The flood carried away photographs and memorabilia going back to grade school, furniture and personal effects of my recently deceased mother, and many of my favorite plants. Although these losses made me sad for a time, oddly, I felt at peace with all of it. To the bewilderment of my partner, who said she couldn't imagine being calm in the face of such news, I declined to return to Arizona, feeling no need to oversee the cleanup and assessment of damage. I was able to let go of attachment to my possessions, and once again, this time in circumstances that I might have expected to make me quite unhappy, I was spontaneously embraced by the feeling that all was as it should be, that my opinions didn't matter, and that I was emotionally free.

Experiences like these give me a sense of emotional well-being, especially in its core elements of resilience and balance. I have already mentioned these factors as defining characteristics of health that allow organisms to interact with potentially harmful influences and not suffer injury or harm. In the emotional realm, resilience enables you to bounce back from losses and reversals and not get stuck in moods that you don't want to be stuck in. Think of an elastic band that can be twisted and stretched but always goes back to its more or less original shape. If you cultivate emotional resilience, you don't have to resist feeling appropriate sadness; you learn that your moods are dynamic and flexible and that they soon return to the neutral balance point, the zone of contentment, comfort, and serenity.

When I ask people to give me images of contentment, they usually come up with ones like these:

- a child licking an ice-cream cone
- a person lying on a couch after a fabulous holiday dinner in the company of family and friends
- a dairy cow munching lush grass in a postcard-perfect meadow
- a dog lying in front of a fire, being stroked by its human companion

I would call these images of satisfaction rather than of contentment, just a temporary response to fulfilling needs or gratifying desires. Contentment, I think, has more to do with being at peace and feeling good about who you are and what you have without regard to satisfying your desires and needs. Contentment is enduring. You carry it with you. The sixth-century BCE Chinese philosopher Lao-tzu got it right (as usual) in few words: "One who contains content, remains content." A striking aspect of this state of mind is that it does not foster passivity (which Westerners often criticize Eastern philosophies for doing). In both 1959 and 2006 and whenever it has returned, my sense that all is right with the world has actually spurred me on to effective action and improved my efficiency.

I suggest that the ability to feel contentment is a key component of emotional well-being. It is also a goal of many religions and philosophies that recognize that the source of human unhappiness is our habit of comparing our experiences to those of others and finding our reality to be wanting. The choice is ours: we can keep on craving what we don't have, and so perpetuate our unhappiness, or we can adjust our attitude toward what we do have so that our expectations conform to our experience. There is much discourse by philosophers and teachers on this theme, because we all eventually learn that we can't always get what we want. How many of us work at appreciating what we have?

If you are not sure what I mean by *work at appreciating what we have,* you will be interested to know that techniques exist for just this kind of practice. They include ancient forms of meditation and new forms of psychotherapy, and I will explain them in chapter 6, where I discuss ways of changing destructive mental habits in order to improve emotional wellness.

What about comfort? The word comes from a Latin root meaning "strength" and denotes a state of ease and freedom from pain and anxiety. To be *comfortable* is to enjoy contentment and security and presumably be stronger as a result. I would argue that, like contentment, comfort is something you can carry with you, a feeling you should be able to access in a great variety of circumstances.

Because I grew up as a city boy and did not live outside an urban environment until my late twenties, I was uncomfortable in nature, unable to enjoy camping or being in the wilderness for more than a few hours. I had to learn how to be at ease in nature, but once I set my mind on doing so, the process was not difficult. It changed me, made me healthier in body and mind, and opened worlds of new experience that have greatly enriched my life. One welcome aspect of the change was that I lost my anxiety around insects, especially bees and wasps, which had made it impossible for me to relax out of doors. I don't know just how this happened, but as it did, I came to understand the behavior of these creatures, appreciate their beauty, and coexist peacefully with them. I've now lived in or near wilderness for most of my adult life and have no problems with insects.

It's good to be comfortable in nature, but it's even more important to be comfortable in your own skin. Whatever your external circumstances, you will not know ease if you are not at ease with yourself. The more comfortable I am with myself, the more effective I am in communicating, teaching, and working with patients, many of whom tell me I am a comforting presence, making it easier for them to talk about their concerns and problems and give me the kind of information I need in order to make accurate diagnoses and determine the best treatment plans.

Serenity is another quality I associate with emotional sea level. We might picture the peaceful calm of still air and an unclouded sky or a placid body of water, but the word *serenity* also refers to the absence of mental stress and anxiety. Again, this emotional state can be cultivated, and maintained, even in the midst of external agitation. A Sufi fable tells of a ship of pilgrims engulfed by a great storm at sea. The passengers are gripped by fear. They wail and moan, sure that death is imminent. Only when the storm subsides do they notice that one of their number, a dervish, has sat through all the tumult in calm meditation. They crowd around him in wonder, and several ask him, "Don't you know that at any moment we could have perished?" He replies, "I know that I might perish at any moment always and have learned to be at peace with that knowledge."

Serenity can be a gift of aging if you are open to it. Many older people tell me they have much greater emotional equilibrium than they did when they were young, that they are better able to adjust to life's ups and downs. Serenity also comes naturally from acceptance, especially of "the things I cannot change," in the words of the much-quoted Serenity Prayer.* But attaining serenity is also a process and a practice. My own efforts to cultivate it through meditation and the practice of nonattachment have had the practical benefit of enabling me to be very cool in emergencies, to respond swiftly and efficiently and not panic, just as I did when my property was flooded.

If you are in good emotional health, you should be able to respond appropriately to whatever situations you encounter: to feel appropriately happy about good fortune and appropriately sad about bad, to be able to feel appropriately angry or frustrated about the state of the

---

* Composed in 1943 by theologian Reinhold Niebuhr.

world and the annoying behavior of others *and to let go of those feelings once you've acknowledged them.* It's important to remember that our moods are supposed to vary through both the positive and negative regions of the emotional spectrum.

Just as we have both cloudy and sunny days, we are all sad at some times and happy at others; such changes are part of dynamic balance. Emotions out of balance are most obvious in individuals with bipolar disorder, marked by the abnormal cycling of mania (elevated mood, energy, and excitement) and depression. Bipolar disorder can cause a great deal of suffering, for both the affected individuals and those around them. Many people with creative talents carry this diagnosis, and some are high achievers, especially in their manic phases, but without treatment, individuals have little chance of maintaining stable relationships or productivity, and the risk of suicide is high. Research on the causes of bipolar disorder suggests that both genetic and environmental factors are involved, and it pinpoints disturbed function in specific brain areas. Management of the disorder relies on psychiatric drugs as well as psychotherapy.

Over the years, a number of bipolar patients have sought my help. Dissatisfied with standard care, especially the side effects of their medications, they have hoped to find ways of being more in control of their erratic moods. In the detailed histories I recorded of them, I noted that the emotional imbalance in these patients always goes along with imbalances in other areas of their lives. Their sleep patterns are erratic, as are their eating, their physical activity, and their ability to maintain order in their living spaces. The essential problem that I perceive in them all is *life out of balance.* The mood disturbances that plague them strike me as exaggerations of normal emotional variability, quantitatively, not qualitatively, different from the changeable moods most of us experience. I would never advise patients with bipolar disorder to discontinue their medication, but I do strongly advise them to cultivate greater balance in their lives wherever they can, by eating at regular times, adhering to a fixed schedule of sleeping and waking, creating order in their physical environments, getting regular exercise, learning yoga or tai chi, and trying some form of meditation. By doing so, they can indirectly improve their emotional health and spend less time at the extremities of the mood spectrum and more toward the midpoint. I follow this advice myself and have incorporated it into the action plan I'll give you in chapter 8.

The mood swings of bipolar disorder exemplify one kind of emotional problem. Just as the variability of the beating of a healthy heart is subtle, so should the variability of human emotions be moderate. It is perfectly normal to experience "the blues," just as it is perfectly normal to experience joy and bliss, but optimizing emotional well-being means gaining greater control of the variability of moods, damping down the oscillations, and enjoying the rewards of the midpoint. It also means not shutting down that dynamic variability, not getting emotionally stuck. Imagine yourself on a seesaw. The goal is to have pleasant excursions around the balance point, not to endure violent swings or to stop moving. And you certainly don't want to get stuck on the ground.

It is near the balance point that you will find resilience, contentment, comfort, and serenity. This is your emotional safe harbor, which you can leave but to which you should be able to return easily and naturally. I advise you to beware of the countless books, websites, television shows, seminars, religions, and drugs (especially drugs) promising ceaseless bliss. The notion that a human being should be constantly happy is a uniquely modern, uniquely American, uniquely destructive idea.

A German friend recently told me that the American greeting ritual — person #1 says, "How are you?" and person #2 must summon a smile and respond, "Great! Great!" — strikes her as bizarre, artificial, and exhausting beyond measure. I agree. I am asked how I am all the time, and as I recite the obligatory "Great!" I can't help wondering what I'm doing. The question feels intrusive, the answer disingenuous, the whole exchange false.

Yet enforced, almost bullying cheerfulness dominates our culture. In her book *Bright-Sided: How the Relentless Promotion of Positive Thinking Has Undermined America,* Barbara Ehrenreich writes that when she was diagnosed with breast cancer in 2000, she found the wildly optimistic pink-ribbon culture surrounding the condition nearly as daunting as the disease itself. It did not allow her to express fear, anger, worry—all perfectly normal responses to a potentially life-threatening diagnosis. Instead she was told over and over that cancer was her chance to grow spiritually, to embrace life, to find God. The message forced on her was "What does not destroy you, [to paraphrase Nietzsche] makes you a spunkier, more evolved sort of person." So put on a happy face.

Ehrenreich goes on to deconstruct the career of George W. Bush, a high school cheerleader (cheerleading, Ehrenreich notes, is an American invention) who maintained that role throughout his presidency, remaining doggedly, destructively optimistic about everything from Wall Street's inability to police itself to America's counterterrorism efforts. "The president almost demanded optimism," noted Bush's secretary of state Condoleezza Rice. "He didn't like pessimism, hand-wringing or doubt." His detractors called this "toxic optimism."

Are we more or less happy than people in other parts of the world? That is not an easy question to answer, in part because different cultures define *happiness* in different ways, and translations of the word might not convey the same meaning. A number of scholarly articles on this subject have appeared in the *Journal of Happiness Studies.* One, from 2004, notes that in Europe and North America, where independence of the self is a cultural norm, happiness is often construed as a positive attribute of the self, to be pursued through personal striving and achievement. In East Asia, on the other hand, happiness is dependent on positive social relationships of which the self is a part; in those cultures, pursuing personal happiness often damages social relationships by creating envy in others, and there is less desire for it. Other scholarly articles report significant differences from country to country in rates of reported happiness, with North Americans at the top, but it is far from clear whether we are actually happier than Germans or Greeks or whether we are just more likely to say we are. (One interesting note is that while the meaning of *happiness* in English has not changed, the adjective *happy* has weakened, so that many people now use it interchangeably with *okay* or *all right*, as in statements like "I'm happy with the new schedule.")

Our cultural insistence on being happy is most obviously counterproductive during the annual holiday season. Throughout most of recorded history, people in the Northern Hemisphere regarded the days around the winter solstice as a time of danger, with the source of light and warmth at its lowest, weakest point in the sky, the months of harshest weather about to come, and a time of short days and long nights, when only the wise could discern the return of the light. The natural cultural response was to gather indoors and huddle in front of fires, feasting together, telling stories, and drawing strength from social bonds. Our culture today, in contrast, tells us that the holiday season is the most wonderful time of the year, when we should all be constantly happy. Bombarded with this message, over and over, at top volume, on all channels so that we cannot escape it, we have developed impossible expectations. The discordance between our expectations of happiness and the emotional realities of the holidays is a major reason for the high incidence of depression at this time of year.

Let me introduce a word that describes a more realistic emotional goal. *Lagom* is a Swedish term that does not have an exact English equivalent; it means something like "just right" or "exactly enough." It has been called the most Swedish of Swedish words, and it permeates the entire culture: architecture, politics, economics, and every aspect of daily life.

Contentment, serenity, comfort, balance, and resilience together constitute a *lagom* version of positive emotionality and, I think, a sane alternative to the perpetual happiness expected and demanded in our society. It should be more than enough to sustain us, and it will not burn us out or condemn us to alternating cycles of bliss and despair. This is what I felt in 1959 and 2006 and at other times in a long and eventful life. I believe it can be cultivated until it becomes our default emotional state. That is what I try to do in my life. It is what this book will help you do in yours.

2

An Epidemic of Depression

"Everyone I know is depressed, including me," says a friend in New York. She adds, "I think the whole country is depressed." These are exaggerations, of course, but statistics indicate that something has gone seriously awry with our emotions. The World Health Organization predicts that by 2030 more people worldwide will be affected by depression than by any other health condition. The number of Americans taking antidepressant drugs doubled in the decade from 1996 to 2005, from 13.3 million to 27 million. Today an astonishing one in ten people in the United States, including millions of children, is on one or more of these medications.

Depression has always been with us, though never so much of it. Ancient Greeks called it *melancholia*, literally meaning "black bile." They believed that a balance of four humors (bodily fluids) affected one's health, with an excess of black bile resulting in sadness. A word of Latin origin for "sad" is *lugubrious*, with a root meaning of "mournful," significant in that depression has long been accepted as a natural response to the loss of a loved one, pathological only when it persists beyond the normal limits of mourning. Lions, some birds, and a few other animals may respond this way to the death of a mate; some lose interest in eating and in caring for themselves and can even die as a result. Some dogs exhibit such behavior when they lose a closely bonded companion, either canine or human.

The sadness of mourning is an example of *situational depression,* a reaction to a terrible loss or other catastrophe, and it makes sense to us, especially if it lifts after an appropriate course of time. But when depression comes for no apparent reason and, worse, refuses to depart, it confounds us. Antonio in Shakespeare's *The Merchant of Venice* complains of causeless sadness—a reflection, some biographers believe, of the playwright's own melancholia:

> *In sooth, I know not why I am so sad:*
> *It wearies me; you say it wearies you;*
> *But how I caught it, found it, or came by it,*
> *What stuff 'tis made of, whereof it is born,*
> *I am to learn....*

Throughout history, people have struggled to account for such *endogenous* (coming from within) *depression.* The distinction between endogenous depression and situational depression still seems useful to me, although the *Diagnostic and Statistical Manual of Mental Disorders* (DSM), published by the American Psychiatric Association, now breaks depression into a great many types and subtypes. The most serious of these is major depressive disorder.

The current edition of the DSM gives specific criteria for the diagnosis of this most severe form of depression. To fall into this category, a patient must have experienced at least one major depressive episode, defined as:

> [A] period of at least 2 weeks during which there is either depressed mood or the loss of interest or pleasure in nearly all activities. In children and adolescents, the mood may be irritable rather than sad. The individual must also experience at least four additional symptoms drawn from a list that includes changes in appetite or weight, sleep, and psychomotor activity; decreased energy; feelings of worthlessness

or guilt; difficulty thinking, concentrating, or making decisions; or recurrent thoughts of death or suicidal ideation, plans or attempts. To count toward a Major Depressive Episode, a symptom must either be newly present or must have clearly worsened compared with the person's pre-episode status. The symptoms must persist for most of the day, nearly every day, for at least 2 consecutive weeks. The episode must be accompanied by clinically significant distress or impairment in social, occupational, or other important areas of functioning.

Major depressive disorder is a serious illness with a high risk of suicide. It always requires competent management by mental health professionals. **The recommendations in this book may be very useful as adjunctive treatments for major depressive disorder, but they should never be used in place of medication or other standard therapy.**

The clinical language of the DSM hardly conveys the suffering of people with severe depression. The novelist William Styron, author of *Sophie's Choice,* provides an eloquent and heartrending interior view of it in his 1990 book, *Darkness Visible: A Memoir of Madness:*

> The pain of severe depression is quite unimaginable to those who have not suffered it.... What I had begun to discover is that, mysteriously and in ways that are totally remote from normal experience, the grey drizzle of horror induced by depression takes on the quality of physical pain. But it is not an immediately identifiable pain, like that of a broken limb. It may be more accurate to say that despair, owing to some evil trick played upon the sick brain by the inhabiting psyche, comes to resemble the diabolical discomfort of being imprisoned in a fiercely overheated room. And because no breeze stirs this cauldron, because there is no escape from the smothering confinement, it is natural that the victim begins to think ceaselessly of oblivion.

I have never felt such lasting emotional pain, nor had a major depressive episode. At various points in my life, however, I have experienced a depressed mood for most of the day more days than not over weeks and even months. During those periods, I also had low energy, feelings of hopelessness, and little desire for social interaction. Sometimes I became anxious and agitated as well. Because my sleep was not refreshing, I found it hard to drag myself out of bed in the morning to face another bleak day of gloomy ruminations about disappointments in life and my own shortcomings. From that emotional vantage point I could see nothing to make me feel cheerful, find nothing to enjoy, no reason to laugh. Luckily, I did not try to boost my mood with alcohol or other substances. (I was aware of the strong association between depression and substance abuse and dependence.) I did turn to food for comfort, often overeating or eating things I normally would not eat, like ice cream and chips.

Some of my most painful memories are of depressions that overcame me when I was living in especially beautiful places. In 1972, for example, I spent a month in a cottage on the shore of Lake Atitlán in the highlands of Guatemala, on my way to South America. The English writer Aldous Huxley wrote of it, "Lake Como [in Italy], it seems to me, touches on the limit of permissibly picturesque, but Atitlán is Como with the additional embellishments of several immense volcanoes. It really is too much of a good thing." In any direction I looked I saw beauty: the deep blue mirrorlike surface of the lake, snowcapped volcanic cones, colorfully dressed Maya Indians on primitive roads that connected their lakeside villages. And I was miserable, unable to shake my dark mood. The contrast between my mood and my surroundings made me feel somehow contaminated and unworthy of the place. Not only did that add to my despair, but it made me even more averse to venturing out and seeking social contact. I told myself that I shouldn't subject others to my negative emotions or risk "infecting" anyone with them.

Over the years I tried various forms of psychotherapy and counseling but got little benefit from them. Once, in my early forties, I filled a prescription for an antidepressant (Zoloft) but gave it up after a few days because I could not tolerate its side effects. It numbed my body and dulled my mind. Although I knew these immediate effects were supposed to pass and I would have had to wait up to several weeks for an improvement in mood, I was unwilling to put up with them.

Eventually I came to accept my depressive episodes as existential in nature—part of my being—to be endured and not inflicted on others. That way of thinking increased my tendency to be antisocial and isolated, traits not uncommon in writers. I even suspected that the introspection associated with these episodes might be a source of creativity and inspiration. (In retrospect, I think social isolation was a major factor in deepening and prolonging my depressions.) This pattern in my emotional life was frequent in my twenties, thirties, and forties, and then it began to wane, and it has steadily diminished and now rarely recurs. When it does, it seldom lasts more than a day or two, even when I encounter tough situations. Possibly, the improvement is a natural reward of aging; more likely, it is the cumulative result of changes I've made in my life. According to the DSM's classification, I would have been diagnosed with dysthymic disorder,* the commonest form of mild to moderate depression. This diagnosis accounts for much of the epidemic of depression occurring today and is the kind most responsive to the interventions suggested in this book.

Dysthymic disorder is distinct from depression associated with psychosis, manic episodes, direct effects of psychoactive drugs or medications, or general medical conditions (like hypothyroidism). The diagnostic criteria for it include a depressed mood for most of the day for more days than not for at least two years, and the presence, while depressed, of two (or more) of the following:

- poor appetite or overeating
- insomnia or hypersomnia (excessive sleep)
- low energy or fatigue
- low self-esteem

---

* *Dysthymia* is derived from Greek roots meaning a "disorder of the mind."

- poor concentration or difficulty making decisions
- feelings of hopelessness

Furthermore, during the two-year period, depressed mood and other symptoms are not absent for more than two months at a time, and they cause clinically significant distress or significant impairment in social, occupational, or other areas of functioning.

I am somewhat wary of trying to classify our emotional states in neat categories as the DSM does, with numerical codes, no less. The DSM puts anxiety disorders in a different section from forms of depression, with different numerical codes, but, as in my case, anxiety often accompanies depression. (A prominent health website notes that in one group surveyed, 85 percent of those with major depressive disorder were also diagnosed with generalized anxiety disorder.) I'm afraid that, despite psychiatry's earnest efforts to emulate the greater precision of other medical specialties, depression cannot easily be packed into diagnostic pigeonholes. It is as protean as the human condition itself. If you suffer from depression, my advice is not to dwell on the DSM's technical descriptions of its various forms, except to make sure that you do not have one that requires professional management and medication, such as major depressive disorder or bipolar disorder. Focus instead on the ways that you can get unstuck emotionally and move the set point of your moods away from depression.

Now to the question I raised at the beginning of this chapter: Why is there an epidemic of depression today? Why are so many people unhappy? What can have changed in our society in the past few decades to account for the unprecedented escalation of depression diagnoses? I say "our society" because, although depression occurs everywhere, nowhere does it affect as many people as in the developed, affluent, technologically advanced countries.

A genetic predisposition has been implicated in depression, but our genes have not changed significantly in the past twenty years.

We know that hormones play a role. Women are twice as likely as men to experience depression; as many as one in four women may suffer a major depressive episode over the course of a lifetime. Before puberty, rates of depression are equal in boys and girls, suggesting that hormonal influences may account for much of the disparity in the adult population. These facts are interesting but do not explain the new trend.

We know also that depression commonly coexists with physical illness: it affects 25 percent of patients with cancer, diabetes, or stroke; 33 percent of heart attack survivors; and 50 percent of those with Parkinson's disease. Many of these chronic conditions are more prevalent today but not prevalent enough to account for so much depression.

Might the epidemic have something to do with the graying of our population in such large numbers, a recent and dramatic change? Older people are more likely to experience bereavement, illness, loss of independence, and other life stresses that can undermine emotional well-being, especially in the absence of strong social support. Nevertheless, experts on aging agree that depression is not a normal consequence of growing older. And one of the age groups most affected lies toward the opposite end of the age spectrum.

The National Institute of Mental Health reports that in any given year, 4 percent of adolescents in our society suffer severe depression. Depression is also being diagnosed much more frequently in preteens than ever before. Along with attention deficit hyperactivity disorder (ADHD) and the autistic disorders, depression accounts for the unprecedented, widespread use of prescribed psychiatric drugs by our young people.

The state of our world is certainly cause for anxiety and gloom, but that is nothing new. In the first half of the twentieth century, a great many people lived through the most horrific wars of all time as well as the worst economic depression, yet they were better off emotionally than many people today. Recall the famous opening lines of Dickens's *A Tale of Two Cities:* "It was the best of times, it was the worst of times, it was . . . the season of Light, it was the season of Darkness, it was the spring of hope, it was the winter of despair, we had everything before us, we had nothing before us…" Such is the state of the world—past, present, and, most likely, future. It is our choice to pay greater attention to its beauty or its ugliness.

Two explanations strike me as most compelling for the present epidemic, and they are by no means mutually exclusive. The first is that a significant portion of the epidemic has been manufactured by the medical-industrial complex. The second is that dramatic changes in living conditions have altered human brain function, dampening emotional variability and displacing its set point toward depression.

Let's examine these one at a time.

To question the legitimacy of the rising incidence of depression diagnoses is provocative and polarizing. But it is undeniable that tremendous profits are being made from the current epidemic—by pharmaceutical companies, big insurers, and corporate health care providers; they all have a huge incentive to keep the epidemic going and growing. Today, direct-to-consumer (DTC) advertising of antidepressant drugs relentlessly pushes the idea that all unhappiness equals depression and is treatable with medication. In 1996, the pharmaceutical industry spent $32 million on DTC antidepressant ads; by 2005, that had nearly quadrupled, to $122 million.

The strategy has certainly worked. More than 164 million antidepressant prescriptions were written in 2008, totaling $9.6 billion in US sales. That's why today, television commercials like this one are ubiquitous:

A morose-looking person stares out of a darkened room through a rain-streaked window. Quick cut to a cheery logo of an SSRI (selective serotonin reuptake inhibitor, the most common type of antidepressant pharmaceutical). Cross-fade to the same person, medicated and smiling, emerging into sunlight to pick flowers, ride a bicycle, or serve birthday cake to laughing children. A voiceover gently suggests, "Ask your doctor if [name of drug] is right for you."

The clear messages are: sadness of any duration is depression;

depression is a chemical imbalance in the brain; and a pill will make you happy — so ask your doctor to prescribe it for you.

Having created a vast American market for antidepressants, drugmakers are now vigorously exporting these dubious messages worldwide. *Crazy Like Us: The Globalization of the American Psyche* by journalist Ethan Watters is a disturbing account of how American psychiatric concepts are displacing traditional cultural views of mental health and illness — especially those surrounding sadness. Mood disorders affect people of all cultures, but their forms of expression vary. A Nigerian man, Watters writes, "might experience a culturally distinct form of depression by describing a peppery feeling in his head. A rural Chinese farmer might speak only of shoulder or stomachaches. A man in India might talk of semen loss or a sinking heart or feeling hot. A Korean might tell you of a 'fire illness' which is experienced as a burning in the gut. Someone from Iran might talk of tightness in the chest, and an American Indian might describe the experience of depression as something akin to loneliness."

Until very recently, the psychiatric term for depression in Japan was *utsubyô,* designating "a mental illness as chronic and devastating as schizophrenia" that makes it impossible to hold a job or have anything like a normal life and requires long-term hospitalization. *Utsubyô* was an uncommon disorder and one surrounded by serious social stigma. It did not offer pharmaceutical companies much opportunity for profit.

Over the past decade, however, a massive marketing campaign launched in Japan by GlaxoSmithKline, makers of Paxil and related SSRI antidepressant drugs, has changed all that. Informed by academic Western psychiatrists about how Japanese concepts of depression differ from those in the United States — and, more to the point, about how those concepts might be transformed — GlaxoSmithKline promoted the idea that depression should be renamed *kokoro no kaze,* meaning something like "a cold of the heart-mind." This new name accomplished three things:

- It implied that depression was not a severe condition and so should not carry a social stigma.
- It suggested that treating depression should be as simple as taking medication for a cold.
- It indicated that, just as everyone got colds from time to time, so did everyone get depressed now and then.

The fact that DTC advertising is illegal in Japan was little impediment; the company pushed this notion in thinly veiled public service announcements on television, as well as in magazine articles, books, and other ostensibly objective media. The result: in 2000, its first year on the Japanese market, Paxil brought in $100 million. By 2008, annual sales in Japan exceeded $1 billion. Asked how he felt about helping drug companies open this market, one American psychiatry professor laughed and remarked, "We were very cheap prostitutes."

Medical doctors, whether in the United States, Japan, or any other country in the pharmaceutical industry's crosshairs, should be a last line of defense against the endless barrage of drug ads and editorial propaganda. After all, none of it would work if physicians refused to prescribe the products.

But physicians *do* prescribe them. Why?

The reality is that the pharmaceutical industry's aggressive marketing meets little resistance from overworked professionals who staff health care systems in much of the developed world. Especially in the United States, physicians often label patients depressed without taking detailed, comprehensive medical histories, and using this diagnosis has become a common and lazy way of handling those with vague or confounding symptoms. Similarly, medicating children frequently takes the place of addressing the complex causes of behavior, learning, and mood disorders—or even unexplained aches and pains. Teens who are grumpy, hostile, or unruly may be judged depressed and put on psychiatric drugs even though they are not sad.

In my view, prescribing antidepressant drugs is too often a quick and easy substitute for developing treatment plans that address the totality of health concerns and lifestyle factors that have an impact on wellness, including emotional wellness. With abbreviated office visits in the current era of managed care and profit-driven medicine, these trends have worsened.

So, then, how much of the depression epidemic is real and how much is spurious? A study published in the April 2007 issue of the *Archives of General Psychiatry* based on a survey of more than eight thousand Americans concluded that estimates of the number who suffer from depression at least once during their lifetimes are about 25 percent too high. The authors noted that the questions clinicians use to determine if patients are depressed don't account for the possibility that they may be reacting *normally* and temporarily to upheavals such as loss of a job or divorce. (Only bereavement due to death is accounted for in the standard clinical assessment.)

Even if much of the current epidemic is manufactured, we are still left with a rise in the incidence of real depression over the past twenty years; indeed, the rate has more than doubled. Not only is it alarmingly high in the United States, but it is also going up in the rest of the developed world, in countries where most people enjoy comfortable lives and the benefits of technology. Despite the comforts and security enjoyed — enviable from the viewpoint of those in less developed areas — there is greater unhappiness.

When I leave modern life behind and travel to those less developed areas, I often encounter less depression and better overall emotional health. I have spent time with people in rural India, Thailand, Latin America, Africa, and the Arctic, and found them to be generally happier and more content than most Americans I know, even though they lack the conveniences and comforts of our advanced society. (Of course, they had food, water, shelter, and security.) Friends and colleagues who have lived in poor countries of the world confirm my impression. Below is an excerpt of a letter I received from Dr. Russell Greenfield, an emergency medicine physician and one of the first graduates of the integrative medicine fellowship of the Arizona Center for Integrative Medicine, which I direct. Russ spent several weeks in Haiti as a volunteer medical worker following the devastating earthquake of January 12, 2010.

I'd like to share a story about a kid (nineteen years old) I helped care for named Junior.

He was on the fourth floor of a building that collapsed and was trapped inside it for days until he was found beneath a couch and refrigerator. When I met Junior weeks after the earthquake, he had lost both legs below the knee and his right arm immediately below the shoulder. Yet every day when I came into the clinic and asked in my broken Creole how he was, he would answer the same way, raising his left arm high into the air and exclaiming as a brilliant smile burst forth, "Great, Dr. Roos!" One day, as we talked at length, Junior told me about his plans to become a minister. Seemingly he had moved on.

I swear that was the way it was for most every patient I cared for. They would open up occasionally and talk about what had transpired but that wasn't their focus. They were looking forward. They had rapidly attained a degree of acceptance I might not have expected in a lifetime, given their circumstances. Instead of obsessing about what had happened to them, they were attending to what they were going to do now. I admired them but was puzzled to the max.

After more than twenty-five years of practicing medicine and with over fifty years of life experience I had confidence in my understanding of human nature; however, my training and previous experience did not prepare me for what I witnessed in Haiti. The people our group ran into had every reason to be depressed and angry, and I expected as much. After all, they had lost loved ones, limbs, their homes and livelihoods, and the days before them were uncertain at best. But they responded not with negative thoughts but with amazing emotional resilience that defied their circumstances. They were full of gratitude for being alive and for what they still had, and repeatedly expressed hope for the future. In the hospital tents, where singing and prayers would break out without warning, their support community actually expanded.

I do not in any way discount the suffering of the Haitian people. I am, however, fascinated by their formidable emotional resilience, as observed by Dr. Greenfield and others.

There is abundant evidence that depression is a "disease of affluence," a disorder of modern life in the industrialized world, even though a recent cross-cultural study suggests that one index of happiness, called "life satisfaction," does increase with income. But the same study reports that the day-to-day sense of how happy one feels ("positive feelings") is almost entirely unconnected to income level. In my experience, the more people have, the less likely they are to be content. Consider the following:

- The risk of developing major depression has increased tenfold since World War II.
- People who live in poorer countries have a lower risk of depression than those in industrialized nations.
- In modernized countries, depression rates are higher for city dwellers than for rural residents.
- In general, countries with lifestyles that are farthest removed from modern standards have the lowest rates of depression.
- Within the United States, the rate of depression among members of the Old Order Amish — a religious sect that shuns modernity in favor of lifestyles roughly emulating those of rural Americans a century ago — is as low as one-tenth that of other Americans.
- Hunter-gatherer societies in the modern world have extremely low rates of depression. The Toraja people of Indonesia, the Trobriand Islanders of Melanesia, and the Kaluli people of Papua New Guinea are examples. Among the thousands of Kaluli assessed for major depressive disorder, a researcher was able to find just one person with the condition.

Psychologist Martin Seligman, originator of the field of positive psychology and director of the Positive Psychology Center at the University of Pennsylvania, has studied the Old Order Amish and the Kaluli. He reports that "neither of these pre-modern cultures has depression at anything like the prevalence we do." And he concludes: "Putting this together, there seems to be something about modern life that creates fertile soil for depression."

Another prominent researcher whose work I respect is Stephen Ilardi, professor of psychology at the University of Kansas and author of *The Depression Cure.* He observes: "The more 'modern' a society's way of life, the higher its rate of depression. It may seem baffling, but the explanation is simple: The human body was never designed for the modern post-industrial environment."

To the extent that the epidemic of depression is real, might it stem from a mismatch between that environment and our genetic heritage? Is it a product of lifestyles strongly influenced by wealth and technology and radically different from those of our parents and grandparents?

I believe so. More and more of us are sedentary, spending most of our time indoors. We eat industrial food much altered from its natural sources, and there is reason for concern about how our changed eating habits are affecting our brain activity and our moods. We are deluged by an unprecedented overload of information and stimulation in this age of the Internet, e-mail, mobile phones, and multimedia, all of which favor social isolation and certainly affect our emotional (and physical) health.

Note that behaviors strongly associated with depression — reduced physical activity and human contact, overconsumption of processed food, a desire for endless distraction — are the very behaviors that more and more people now *can* indulge in, or are even forced to embrace by the nature of their sedentary indoor jobs.

This kind of life simply was not an option throughout most of human history, as there was no infrastructure to support it, much less require it. No one on earth is that far from a hunter-gatherer lifestyle chronologically. Agriculture began ten thousand years ago, and as recently as 1801, 95 percent of Americans still lived on farms. By 1901, the figure was 45 percent; by the turn of the twenty-first century, less than 2 percent. And before the advent of industrial agriculture, farmers lived far healthier lives than most of us today. Lacking the benefits of modern medicine and advancements in public health, they were at greater risk of infectious disease, but they spent much more time outdoors and in nature, conditioned their bodies with integrative exercise from manual labor, ate wholesome food, communicated with others face-to-face, and enjoyed the social support of rural communities.

Seligman, Ilardi, and I are not arguing that life for our ancestors or modernity-shunning contemporaries was (or is) easy. Indeed, it was often quite arduous in ways we can scarcely imagine today. But *hard* does not mean *depressed,* just as *easy* does not mean *content.* In fact, hard lives such as those of our ancestors and our "primitive" contemporaries seem to keep the human emotional set point better adjusted. To state a complex change simply: our lives in the developed world have largely gone from *hard* and *generally content* to *easy* and *often depressed.*

Human beings evolved to thrive in natural environments and in bonded social groups. Few of us today can enjoy such a life and the emotional equilibrium it engenders, but our genetic predisposition for it has not changed. The term *nature deficit disorder* has recently entered the popular vocabulary, though it has not yet made it into the DSM or been accepted by the medical community. It was coined a few years ago* to explain a wide range of behavior problems in children who spend little time outdoors, and now it is invoked as the root cause of an even wider range of ailments both physical and emotional in people of all ages who are disconnected from nature.

I believe we are gathering scientific evidence for the benefits of living close to nature, not simply for enjoying its beauty or getting

---

* Richard Louv used it first in his book *Lost Child in the Woods* (2005).

spiritual sustenance, but also for keeping our brains and nervous systems in good working order. A few examples:

- We get vitamin D, now known to be necessary for optimum brain health, by spending time in the sun.
- Our cycles of sleep and waking and other circadian rhythms are maintained by exposure to bright light during the day and darkness at night. Lack of bright natural light during waking hours and exposure to artificial light at night disrupt these rhythms, interfering with our sleep, energy, and moods.
- Hunter-gatherers and other "primitive" peoples do not develop the deficits of vision and the need for corrective lenses as early in life as people in our society do, probably because they grow up looking at distant landscapes more often than reading books, writing, or staring at television and computer screens. Because the eye is a direct extension of the brain, eye health is an indicator of brain health.
- Our hearing has evolved to attend to and analyze changes in the complex acoustical patterns of nature, like those of forests, running water, rain, and wind. Evolution did not prepare us to endure the kinds of man-made sounds that pervade our cities and lives today. Noise strongly affects our emotions, nervous systems, and physiology. I identify it as a major cause of anxiety.

The problems stemming from nature deficit disorder are examples of a mismatch between our genes and the modern environment. Our brains simply are not suited for the modern world. Possibly, the deterioration of emotional well-being characteristic of contemporary urban life represents a cumulative effect of lifestyle changes that have been occurring over many years, an effect that is now suddenly obvious. Still, I wonder which changes in particular might account for the dramatic increase in depression of the past twenty years. Urbanization and disconnection from nature have been going on for a long time. The proliferation of industrial food has happened over just the past fifty years, but I doubt that it is chiefly to blame. If I were to single out one recent change, I would point to the revolutionary new technologies of communication and information delivery, which I believe are altering the activity of our brains and driving our social isolation. Not only do we suffer from nature deficit, but we are also experiencing information surfeit. Many people today spend much of their waking time surfing the Internet, texting and talking on mobile phones, attending to e-mail, watching television, and being stimulated by other new media—all experiences that were unavailable until recently. I believe that all of this stimulation, unprecedented both in kind and in amount, is a major challenge to emotional well-being and likely a significant factor in the current epidemic of depression.

As people become more prosperous, they become more isolated. Material abundance persuades us that we don't really need groups of intimates (and all of the inevitable interpersonal conflicts that come with large families or tribes). Before people could afford to buy air conditioners, for instance, they spent hot summer evenings on front stoops and porches and in town squares, socializing with neighbors. (I remember that well from my childhood in a row house in Philadelphia.) Air-conditioning and other modern conveniences allow us to stay indoors by ourselves. "Now I can take care of myself," we say, thinking that is a good thing. Meanwhile, the allure of synthetic entertainment—television, the Internet—is eerily reminiscent of the false promise of industrial food. It seems like a distillation of the good aspects of a social life—always entertaining yet easy to abandon when it becomes tedious or challenging. But, like junk food, it is ultimately unsatisfying and potentially harmful. Our brains, genetically adapted to help us negotiate a successful course through complex, changing, and often hazardous natural environments, are suddenly confronted with an overload of information and stimulation independent of physical reality.

And here we are. More of us than ever are depressed. The only solution I see is to adjust our lifestyles, not by becoming farmers, hunter-gatherers, or cavemen, but by adapting the healthy habits and behaviors of those people to the context of the modern world. To prevent and treat depression and attain optimum emotional well-being, we have to eat and exercise properly, but we also have to attend to the ways we use our minds and work at reducing distraction and social isolation. I will give you the specifics in part 2 of this book.

Before I leave the subject of depression, I want to look at it from one other perspective, that of the relatively new field of evolutionary psychology, which seeks to explain our psychological traits as adaptations or functional products of natural selection. In describing my own experiences of depression, I wrote that I thought the intense introspection associated with them was somehow a source of inspiration. I felt that going inward so deeply, even in such negative moods, allowed me access to creative energy otherwise out of reach. As I mentioned, many highly creative, accomplished people have struggled with depression. If I were to name all of the writers, artists, composers, and performers affected by it, the list would indeed be very long. Many have become addicted to alcohol or mood-altering drugs, and not a few have committed suicide.

More than twenty studies support a link between depression and creativity. Possibly, writers, artists, and other creative people are more driven to understand themselves and so turn their minds inward, mulling possibilities, seeking answers, and mentally exploring what's wrong and how it might be set right. A word for this mental process is *rumination,* usually considered an aspect of the pathology of depression. To *ruminate* is "to think again and again, to muse, to contemplate, to ponder." Clinical psychologists see rumination as a "way of responding to distress that involves repetitively focusing on the symptoms of distress, and on its possible causes and consequences." But rumination also seems to be exactly the focused interior mental process that underlies creativity. Might it, and even the human susceptibility to depression, serve a purpose from an evolutionary perspective?

Andy Thomson, a psychiatrist at the University of Virginia, and Paul Andrews, an evolutionary psychologist at Virginia Commonwealth University, have suggested an answer to this question, as described in a 2010 *New York Times Magazine* article titled "Depression's Upside."

> [The two investigators] started with the observation that rumination was often a response to a specific psychological blow, like the death of a loved one or the loss of a job. (Darwin was plunged into a debilitating grief after his ten-year-old daughter, Annie, died following a bout of scarlet fever.) Although the DSM manual, the diagnostic bible for psychiatrists, does not take such stressors into account when diagnosing depressive disorder—the exception is grief caused by bereavement, if the grief lasts longer than two months—it's clear that the problems of everyday life play a huge role in causing mental illness. "Of course, rumination is unpleasant," Andrews says. "But it's usually a response to something real, a real setback. It didn't seem right that the brain would go haywire just when we need it most."
>
> Imagine, for instance, a depression triggered by a bitter divorce. The ruminations might take the form of regret ("I should have been a better spouse"), recurring counterfactuals ("What if I hadn't had my affair?") and anxiety about the future ("How will the kids deal with it? Can I afford my alimony payments?"). While such thoughts reinforce the depression—that's why therapists try to stop the ruminative cycle—Andrews and Thomson wondered if they might also help people prepare for bachelorhood or allow people to learn from their mistakes. "I started thinking about how, even if you are depressed for a few months, the depression might be worth it if it helps you better understand social relationships," Andrews says. "Maybe you realize you need to be less rigid or more loving. Those are insights that can come out of depression, and they can be very valuable."

Like Thomson and Andrews, as I wrote in the introduction to this book, I believe that it may be normal, healthy, and even productive to experience mild to moderate depression from time to time as part of the variable emotional spectrum, either as an appropriate response to situations or as a way of turning inward and mentally chewing over problems to find solutions. I still value my occasional periods of depressed mood as sources of intuitive knowledge, inspiration, and creative energy, and when I come out of them, I feel more vital and am more productive. I have found strategies to help me get through them, and I'm much relieved that I no longer get stuck in them.

The poet John Keats wrote in a letter, "Do you not see how necessary a World of Pains and troubles is to school an Intelligence and make it a soul?" But I am hesitant to go too far in justifying or romanticizing depression. It may yield fruit that is worth occasional emotional pain, but no one, I believe, benefits from months or years of sadness, self-loathing, and endlessly cycling rumination. I am sure that most people caught up in the present epidemic of depression want to be free of it. The best way to achieve that is to understand and address all of the factors within our control that influence our emotional resilience and set point. Read on: I will tell you how to do that as soon as I explain the old and new ways of understanding and influencing the relationship between the activity of our brains and our emotions. I assure you that it's possible. You can get there.

3

The Need for a New Approach to Mental Health

Epidemic depression is occurring at a time when the field of mental health appears very robust. There are more mental health professionals treating more people than ever before in history: psychiatrists, clinical psychologists, licensed social workers, counselors, and therapists of all kinds. We have a powerful "therapeutic arsenal" of drugs to make us happier, calmer, and saner. When I leaf through the pharmaceutical ads that take up so much space in psychiatric journals, I get the feeling that we should all be in great emotional health. Depression and anxiety should be as fully conquered as smallpox and polio. But more of us than ever are discontented and not experiencing optimum emotional well-being. What is wrong with this picture? Why is the vast enterprise of professional mental health unable to help us feel better?

I want you to consider the possibility that the basic assumptions of mainstream psychiatric medicine are obsolete and no longer serve us well. Those assumptions constitute the biomedical model of mental health and dominate the whole field.

In 1977, the journal *Science* published a provocative article titled "The Need for a New Medical Model: A Challenge for Biomedicine." I consider it a landmark in medical philosophy and the intellectual foundation of today's integrative medicine. The author, George L. Engel, MD, was a professor of psychiatry at the University of Rochester (New York) School of Medicine. Determined to overcome the limiting influence of Cartesian dualism, which assigns mind and body to separate realms, Engel envisioned medical students of the future learning that health and illness result from an interaction of biological, psychological, social, and behavioral factors, not from biological factors alone. He fathered the field of psychosomatic medicine and devoted much of his career to broadening our understanding of disease. He was particularly interested in mental health.

George Engel died in 1999 with his vision largely unrealized. In fact, the field of psychosomatic medicine ran out of steam sometime before his death and was never able to challenge the ascendancy of biological medicine.

"Biology Explains All" was in full swing when I was a student at Harvard Medical School in the late 1960s. At that time, I was taught that just four diseases were psychosomatic: peptic ulcer, rheumatoid arthritis, bronchial asthma, and ulcerative colitis. Four out of the entire catalog of diseases is not a lot, but at least for those four, doctors conceded that mental/emotional factors played a role. Peptic ulcer was knocked off the list in the early 1980s when a bacterial infection *(Helicobacter pylori)* was identified as the "real" cause of ulcers, now treatable with antibiotics. Investigation of biological factors associated with the three remaining conditions has led to more powerful drug treatments for them and greatly lessened interest in attending to any psychological, social, or behavioral factors that might be involved. Rheumatologists today, for example, are most enthusiastic about a new class of immunosuppressive drugs called TNF-α blockers,* which often appear to put rheumatoid arthritis and ulcerative colitis into full remission. Never mind that these drugs can be highly toxic and are very expensive; once

---

* For "tumor necrosis factor-alpha," a chemical messenger of the immune system; Remicade (infliximab) is a popular one.

doctors prescribe them for these conditions, they no longer see the point of addressing emotional or lifestyle factors of the patients who have them.

Although George Engel's efforts in psychosomatic medicine were ahead of their time, their relevance today is great, and I advise all health professionals, especially mental health professionals, to read his 1977 paper in *Science*. I will summarize his "challenge for biomedicine" here, because it exposes the great limitations of the conceptual model that now dominates medicine in general and psychiatric medicine in particular. That model often fails to help doctors maintain and heal our physical bodies, and it has greatly hindered our understanding of and ability to manage the epidemic of depression and other mood disorders that plague our society. It does not point the way to contentment, comfort, serenity, and resilience, nor does it show us how to attain optimum emotional well-being.

Models are belief systems — sets of assumptions and explanations we construct to make sense of our experience. In Engel's words, "The more socially disruptive or individually upsetting the phenomenon, the more pressing the need of humans to devise explanatory systems." Disease is a very upsetting phenomenon, and humans throughout history have come up with a variety of belief systems to explain it, from the wrath of the gods to possession by spirits to disharmony with the forces of nature. The dominant model of disease in our time is biomedical, built on a foundation of molecular biology. As Engel explains,

> It assumes disease to be fully accounted for by deviations from the norm of measurable biological (somatic) variables. It leaves no room within its framework for the social, psychological, and behavioral dimensions of illness. The biomedical model not only requires that disease be dealt with as an entity independent of social behavior, it also demands that behavioral aberrations be explained on the basis of disordered somatic (biochemical or neurophysiological) processes. Thus the biomedical model embraces both reductionism, the philosophic view that complex phenomena are ultimately derived from a single primary principle, and mind-body dualism.

Engel goes on to say, "The biomedical model has...become a cultural imperative, its limitations easily overlooked. In brief, it has now acquired the status of a *dogma*.... Biological dogma requires that all disease, including 'mental' disease, be conceptualized in terms of derangement of underlying physical mechanisms." He proposed an alternative: a *biopsychosocial* model of health and illness.

There is no question that over the past century, biomedicine has advanced our knowledge of human biology, but the real test of a scientific model—the measure of its superiority to an alternative belief system—is whether or not it increases our ability to describe, predict, and control natural phenomena. In my books about health and healing, I have written a great deal about how strict application of the biomedical model has actually made it harder for us to understand and manage common diseases. For instance, I have pointed out that it fails to account for the fact that many people infected with *H. pylori* never develop peptic ulcers or have any symptoms at all. They coexist with it in a balanced way. Clearly, factors other than the simple presence of that germ play a role in peptic ulcer disease, including the strength or weakness of host defenses, of an individual's resistance. One of those defenses is stomach acid, whose production is influenced by the autonomic (involuntary) nervous system and through it by emotions. In the fight-or-flight response, the sympathetic division of the autonomic nervous system shuts down gastrointestinal function, which is unnecessary in an emergency, in order to divert energy and blood flow to muscles. That includes turning off the production of acid in the stomach. In chronic anxiety and stress, the sympathetic nerves are constantly overactive, and therefore there is constantly less acid in the stomach to keep potentially invasive germs from causing tissue damage. To say that *H. pylori* infection is strongly correlated with peptic ulcer disease is accurate. To say that it is the sole cause of ulcers ignores the complexity of causation and the possible influence of emotions.

In 1980, the American Psychiatric Association radically revised the *Diagnostic and Statistical Manual-III* (DSM-III) to be in accord with the biomedical model. As a consequence, the role of psychiatrists went from being facilitators of insight in patients to being dispensers of drugs to modify brain chemistry. Although some psychiatrists still rely on talk therapy, of all medical specialties, the profession as a whole is the most dominated and, to my mind, hobbled by blind faith in biomedicine. Psychiatrists were easily seduced because of a collective inferiority complex with regard to their place in the medical hierarchy. Still referred to as witch doctors and shrinks (from headshrinkers), they themselves have a history of questioning whether they are real doctors and whether they need the same basic medical training as cardiologists and surgeons. With the spectacular rise of biomedicine, their discomfort increased, and, not wanting to be left behind, they looked for ways to be even more biologically correct than their colleagues in other specialties. They saw their ticket to acceptance in the new and rapidly developing field of psychopharmacology—the study of the effect of drugs on mental and emotional disorders.

In 1921, Otto Loewi (1873–1961), a German pharmacologist, demonstrated that nerve cells (neurons) communicate by releasing chemicals. Prior to that time, neuroscientists thought nervous communication was electrical. Among the many important breakthroughs that followed from Loewi's work were the identification of neurotransmitters and the discovery of receptors on cell surfaces that bind them. Neurotransmitters are chemicals made within the body, stored in tiny sacs clustered within a neuron and released into the synapse, the gap between the neuron and a target cell, which might be another neuron (the postsynaptic neuron) or a muscle or glandular cell. The released molecules then bind to receptors—specialized proteins on the surface membrane of the target cell—causing changes in that cell, making it more or less likely to produce an electrical signal (in the case of a neuron), to contract (in the case of a muscle), or to secrete a hormone (in the case of a glandular cell). Later, the neurotransmitters can separate from their receptors and be taken up by presynaptic cells for reuse or be broken down by enzymes into inactive metabolites. Neuroscientists have now compiled long lists of neurotransmitters, described their actions, and identified many types and subtypes of receptors.

Three of the most studied neurotransmitters are norepinephrine, dopamine, and serotonin, all very relevant to the subject matter of this book because they influence our moods and emotions. For example, dopamine is involved in what is known as the reward system of the brain; drugs that affect it can alter our experience of pleasure. Cocaine is such a drug. It blocks reuptake of dopamine back into the presynaptic neuron, effectively increasing its action at the synapse to produce an intense pleasurable response. With prolonged use of cocaine, postsynaptic neurons become less responsive to dopamine, leading to depression and dependence on the drug to relieve it. The dopamine hypothesis of schizophrenia attributes psychosis to overactivity of this neurotransmitter. Norepinephrine regulates both reward and arousal. Disturbances in that neurotransmitter system are associated with anxiety disorders. And serotonin affects our moods and sleep.

The most widely used psychiatric drugs today influence the production and effects of these major neurotransmitters. Psychopharmacologists made their first big breakthrough in the 1950s from work with antihistamines, used to quell allergic symptoms. Although antihistamines are best known for blocking the effects of the compound responsible for certain immune responses, they also affect the brain, often making people groggy, sleepy, and depressed. By tinkering with these molecules, chemists produced a new class of psychoactive drugs — the phenothiazines — that blocked dopamine transmission. Thorazine and other phenothiazines were successfully marketed as major tranquilizers and antipsychotics and quickly revolutionized the treatment of schizophrenia. Psychiatrists hailed them as magical compounds that cured psychosis, while critics argued that they simply made psychotic people groggy, sedated, and easier to manage, even as outpatients. Energized by this achievement, psychopharmacologists then turned their attention to depression. Over the past sixty years, they have come up with a number of drugs to treat it.

The efforts of psychopharmacologists give us an opportunity to evaluate the usefulness of the biomedical model in psychiatry. In practice, psychiatric medicine today is synonymous with psychopharmacology. The credo of that field is "There is no twisted thought without a twisted molecule."* The biomedical model explains depression as the result of a chemical imbalance in the brain, specifically of neurotransmitters affecting our moods. How well does that explanation enable us to describe, predict, and control depressive illness? In other words, just how effective are the antidepressant drugs that psychopharmacologists have developed, that the big pharmaceutical companies sell such quantities of, and that so many people today take? The answer, I'm afraid, is not very.

The first antidepressant drug was discovered serendipitously in 1952. Iproniazid, an antimicrobial agent being studied as a possible treatment for tuberculosis, was found to affect mood, making even terminally ill patients cheerful and optimistic. Investigation of a possible mechanism for this unexpected psychoactivity revealed that the drug blocked enzymatic breakdown of all three major neurotransmitters: norepinephrine, dopamine, and serotonin. Pharmaceutical chemists then looked for other drugs with this action and soon after produced a different class of antidepressant drugs by modifying the phenothiazine tranquilizers. These became known as tricyclic antidepressants, of which amitriptyline was the prototype; Merck pharmaceutical company gave it the brand name Elavil. In 1961, the FDA approved Elavil for the treatment of major depression, and it quickly became a bestselling drug. The tricyclics appeared to work by blocking presynaptic reuptake of norepinephrine and serotonin without affecting dopamine.

Because all of the early antidepressants had unpleasant side effects and serious potential interactions with other drugs and medications, pharmaceutical chemists continued their search for better ones with more specific action. But what specific action should it be? Some thought deficiency of norepinephrine was the biochemical cause of

---

* The words of the American neurophysiologist Ralph Gerard (1900–1974).

depression. Others argued for a serotonin hypothesis of depression and looked for compounds to prevent its breakdown or reuptake. The proponents of the serotonin hypothesis would win the day; their big discovery came in the 1970s, again, interestingly enough, as a result of work with an antihistamine.

Very likely you have taken Benadryl (diphenhydramine) at some point in your life. It is one of the oldest and most widely used antihistamines, the first such drug to be approved by the FDA for prescription use.* Benadryl is so sedating that it is now sold over the counter as a sleep aid. In the 1960s, this tried-and-true drug was found to have an action independent of its effect on histamine: it selectively inhibited the reuptake of serotonin. By modifying this molecule, scientists at Eli Lilly and Company in the 1970s came up with the first safe and effective selective serotonin reuptake inhibitor, fluoxetine, much better known by its brand name Prozac. The rest is history. Today the accepted biomedical explanation of depression is that it results from a deficiency of serotonin at synapses in key areas of the brain; therefore, boosting the activity of this neurotransmitter with drugs that block its reuptake will treat or cure the problem.

It's a good bet that thirty years ago, not one American in a thousand had heard of this neurotransmitter—or any neurotransmitters, for that matter. Today, when you Google *serotonin,* about 11 million results appear, and Amazon sells nearly three thousand books with the word in the title (including *The Serotonin Solution: The Potent Brain Chemical That Can Help You Stop Bingeing, Lose Weight, and Feel Great*). "Serotonin" is the name of a professional wrestling team and an album by the British rockers The Mystery Jets. You can even proclaim your autumn blues to friends by way of a greeting card that reads, "The leaves and my serotonin levels are falling." A once-obscure neurochemical has become pop-culture currency, and increasing levels of this feelgood compound has turned into a public obsession.

---

* In 1946.

None of this just happened on its own. In order to sell antidepressant medications, drug manufacturers launched a relentless worldwide marketing and public-relations campaign promoting serotonin as the distilled biochemical essence of happiness. The message was that selective serotonin reuptake inhibitors—SSRIs—increase synaptic levels of serotonin in the brain by slowing its rate of reabsorption by presynaptic neurons, ending depression. Psychiatrists and other physicians got the technical version of this message, while consumers got a simplified one, often reduced to the rallying cry "Boost serotonin!"

The only problem is that it probably isn't true.

Like the dopamine hypothesis of schizophrenia and other attempts to attribute complex mental phenomena to simplistic biochemical causes, the serotonin hypothesis of depression is shaky at best. Several studies have established that lowering serotonin levels does *not* negatively impact mood. In fact, a new pharmaceutical known as tianeptine—sold in France and other European countries under the trade name Coaxil—has been shown to be as effective as Prozac. Tianeptine works by *lowering* synaptic serotonin. As psychology professor Irving Kirsch of the University of Hull in England told *Newsweek,* "If depression can be equally affected by drugs that increase serotonin and by drugs that decrease it, it's hard to imagine how the benefits can be due to their chemical activity."

It is, indeed, especially as evidence accumulates that, in most cases, SSRIs work no better than placebos to boost mood. The first such analysis, published in 1998, looked at thirty-eight manufacturer-sponsored studies that included more than three thousand depressed patients. It found negligible differences in improvement between those on the drugs and those on dummy pills. At least 75 percent of the benefit from this class of antidepressants seemed to be a placebo effect. This finding has since been confirmed by other research.

To say that biomedically minded physicians have been reluctant to accept this finding or modify their prescribing habits as a result would be a great understatement. Both professional and popular media have tried to play down the significance of this new research and in some cases have misreported the findings. In April 2002, the *Journal of the American Medical Association (JAMA)* published the results of a large randomized controlled study sponsored by the National Institutes of Health to evaluate a popular herbal treatment for depression, St. John's wort *(Hypericum perforatum)*. Its effect was compared with that of the widely prescribed SSRI Zoloft (sertraline) and a placebo in 340 patients with major depressive disorder. The conclusion that made front-page news around the world was that St. John's wort worked no better than the placebo at relieving depression. Television news shows featured reporters in health-food stores pointing to St. John's wort products and advising consumers not to waste their money on natural remedies whose supposed benefits were nothing more than old wives' tales.

Never mind that St. John's wort is not indicated for the treatment of major depression, making the point of the study questionable. (There is evidence that it is useful in mild to moderate depression, and I'll tell you about that in chapter 5.) The finding from this well-designed trial that should have made front-page news was that Zoloft also worked no better than the placebo. In fact, the placebo treatment was actually more effective in these very depressed patients than either Zoloft or St. John's wort!

Irving Kirsch summarized the growing body of evidence against SSRIs in his 2010 book, *The Emperor's New Drugs: Exploding the Antidepressant Myth,* which I recommend. In response, proponents of the drugs and the serotonin hypothesis retreated to a more defensible position: SSRIs may owe much of their apparent benefit to patients' belief in them, they admit, but they still have a real biochemical effect that makes them useful in the treatment of *severe* depression. Unfortunately for those proponents, the most recent analysis, published in the January 6, 2010, issue of *JAMA,* rates the real biochemical effect of SSRIs as nonexistent to negligible even in most cases of severe depression. Only in patients with very severe symptoms can researchers detect a statistically significant drug benefit compared with that of a placebo. About 13 percent of people with depression have very severe symptoms. One of the authors of the *JAMA* paper, Steven D. Hollon, PhD, of Vanderbilt

University, has said, "Most people [with depression] don't need an active drug. For a lot of folks, you're going to do as well on a sugar pill or on conversations with your physicians as you will on medication. It doesn't matter what you do; it's just that you're doing something."

I would argue that the dismal performance of Prozac, Zoloft, Paxil, and other antidepressant drugs relative to placebos not only leaves the serotonin hypothesis of depression without a leg to stand on but also exposes the failure of the biomedical model to further our understanding of and ability to manage emotional disorders. I firmly believe that the nature of depression will never be revealed solely in studies of brain biochemistry that are isolated from the rest of human experience. Like coronary heart disease, depression is a multifactorial health problem, rooted in complex interactions of biological, psychological, and social variables, best understood and managed through a broader biopsychosocial model of the sort proposed by George Engel.

Loneliness, for example, is a powerful predictor of depression. Numerous studies show that people with few intimate social contacts are more likely to be depressed than those who enjoy a rich network of friends and family. Reductionists might argue that being part of a social group boosts serotonin, but I am confident that there is something in a successful social life that transcends any effect on brain biochemistry, at least insofar as we currently understand that biochemistry. In other words, a happy family life probably raises serotonin in some people, lowers it in others, and leaves it unaffected in still others. Yet it makes them all more comfortable, serene, and relatively immune to mood disorders through a body-mind-social interaction that can't be reduced to its constituent parts.

THE NEW MODEL

In chapter 2 I wrote about possible causes of epidemic depression in our society, among them such lifestyle factors as diets high in processed foods, lack of physical activity, social isolation resulting from affluence, and altered brain activity from information overload. In its narrow focus on molecular biology, the biomedical model fails to capture any of this, and practitioners under its spell cannot give depressed patients the advice they need to address the complex causes of their problems. All they can do is dispense drugs that for the majority of patients might as well be sugar pills.

In an effort to give mental health professionals more and better options, I convened the first national conference on integrative mental health in March 2010. Together with Victoria Maizes, MD, executive director of the Arizona Center for Integrative Medicine, I invited psychiatrists, psychologists, social workers, and other health professionals to attend a three-day event in Phoenix to "learn how to treat their patients within a new paradigm of integrative mental health care that utilizes scientifically proven alternative methods in combination with drugs and traditional therapy to address patients' physical, psychological, and spiritual needs." The use of the word *spiritual* here is significant; it expands George Engel's concept to include yet another dimension of human life, one often overlooked in medicine. Adding it creates a biopsychosocialspiritual model. For convenience, I prefer the term *integrative* to describe this new way of thinking about health and illness in general and mental health in particular.

Dr. Maizes and I invited leading practitioners and researchers to share their experience and findings with attendees. We planned for an audience of three hundred, but, in a time of great economic recession, the conference sold out six weeks in advance with a total of seven hundred registrants. If we had had a larger venue, we could have doubled that number, so great was the interest in the topic—evidence, I think, that professionals are even more fed up than patients with the dead end that the drug-only approach represents.

On the closing day of the conference, I spoke about the failure of the biomedical model and the great advantages of the new integrative model of mental health. I quoted Albert Einstein on the subject of conceptual models:

> Creating a new theory is not like destroying an old barn and erecting a skyscraper in its place. It is rather like climbing a mountain, gaining new and wider views, discovering unexpected connections between our starting point and its rich environment. But the point from which we started still exists and can be seen, although it appears smaller and forms a tiny part of our broad view gained by the mastery of the obstacles on our adventurous way up.

The new integrative model of mental health does not ignore brain biochemistry. It takes into account correlations between imbalances in neurotransmitters and mood disorders. Nor does it reject psychopharmacology. Integrative treatment plans for depression, particularly for severe depression, may well include medication, but my colleagues and I prefer to try other methods first and to use antidepressant drugs for short-term management of crises rather than rely on them as long-term solutions. (In chapter 5, I'll tell you when and how I recommend using them.) One of the invited speakers, a noted expert on psychopharmacology, gave an optimistic presentation on psychiatric drugs of the future, drugs that will have more specific, better-targeted actions. People listened to his lecture with interest but showed much greater enthusiasm for talks on the critical importance of dietary omega-3 fatty acids to optimum emotional health and the latest neuroscientific evidence for the benefits of meditation, among others.

Here's a sampling of the presentations:

- Nutritional Management of Bipolar Disorder in Adults and Youth
- Laughter Therapy
- Mind-Body Medicine — Clinical Hypnosis for Medical and Mental Health Conditions

- Creating the Chemistry of Joy: Integrating Natural and Mindfulness Therapies for Anxiety and Depression
- Acupuncture and Chinese Medicine for Mental Health
- Transforming Your Mind by Changing Your Brain: Meditation and Neuroplasticity
- Deficiencies in Omega-3 Essential Fatty Acids and Mechanisms of Substance Abuse
- Sleep, Dreams, and Mental Health: A Critical Link

To say that the psychiatrists, psychologists, and other mental health professionals in attendance appreciated this larger perspective fails to convey their excitement. One told me that she had been waiting years for such a conference. Another said he would take the information he received and use it to change standards of practice in a large group of mental health care facilities in his state. Many expressed interest in seeking formal training in integrative mental health, training that I and my colleagues at the University of Arizona hope to provide. Dr. Ulka Agarwal, head psychiatrist at the California State University East Bay student health center, wrote me:

> I recently saw a twenty-five-year-old female with moderate depression. She had a bad experience with antidepressants in the past and did not want to try another one. She could not afford counseling and did not have much direction or social support in her life. She asked me about making dietary changes and was thinking about buying supplements she saw on TV. I felt she needed some intervention and she was very open to trying natural treatments, but I didn't know how to advise her. I was really disappointed, and clearly she was too. This was one time too many that a client was willing to make lifestyle changes, yet I did not have the knowledge to help them. I am very excited to be trained in integrative mental health and finally be able to offer my patients the guidance and information they need to start feeling better.

Presentations that particularly interested me concerned neuroplasticity, the potential of the brain and nervous system to change and adapt. The speakers were neuroscientists influenced by Buddhist psychology and the teachings of the Dalai Lama.* Using such new techniques as PET scans and functional MRIs, which make it possible to visualize living brains, they have been able to show that individuals trained in meditation have different brain activity from those without such training, and they respond differently to situations that would cause most of us to lose our emotional equilibrium. The broader implication of this research is that changes in the mind can *cause* changes in both the function and structure of the brain, a fact that cannot be explained by the biomedical model and that suggests many more options for taking charge of our emotional well-being.

In retrospect, seeing human beings as nothing more than the sum of biochemical interactions was probably a necessary stage of medical evolution. Medical systems of the past lacked the technology to study the biological underpinnings of human health with rigor and precision. Now we have that technology, and we've used it well to gain invaluable insights about our physical bodies. But it is impossible to restore or promote human health unless we begin with a complete definition of a human being. An incomplete definition will always result in incomplete diagnoses and less-than-optimal treatments.

So now is the time to ascend the mountain and see the biomedical model as one part of our broadening view. Our health or lack of it is the result of biochemical interactions *and* genetics, dietary choices, exercise patterns, sleep habits, hopes, fears, families, friends, jobs, hobbies, cultures, ecosystems, and more. Chemical imbalances in the brain may well correlate with depression, anxiety, and other emotional

---

* Richard Davidson, PhD, director of the Laboratory for Affective Neuroscience and the Waisman Laboratory for Brain Imaging and Behavior, University of Wisconsin–Madison; Jon Kabat-Zinn, PhD, founder of the Stress Reduction Clinic and Center for Mindfulness in Medicine, Health Care and Society, University of Massachusetts Medical School; Daniel Siegel, MD, of the Mindful Awareness Research Center, UCLA School of Medicine.

disturbances, but the arrows of cause and effect can point in both directions. Optimizing emotional wellness, as by improving attention, changing destructive patterns of thinking, and finding contentment within, can also optimize brain chemistry, correcting any deficiencies in neurotransmitters.

George Engel showed us the path upward more than thirty years ago. Now, I am happy to say, we are starting to follow it.

4

Integrating Eastern and Western Psychology

As a lifelong medical multiculturalist, I've always tried to combine the best ideas and methods of contemporary scientific medicine with those of traditional systems of healing, some of which have their origins in the distant past. I find this approach particularly useful when it comes to mental health. Today's mental health practitioners know a great deal about the brain and mind; traditional psychological knowledge is different but just as impressive. Ancient peoples did not have the scientific tools to investigate neuroanatomy and brain biochemistry, but they desired serenity and freedom from emotional pain as much as we do. Whereas Western science has examined mental phenomena objectively, traditional "researchers," especially in Eastern cultures, used their own minds as laboratories and learned to manipulate subjective experience to achieve desired outcomes. The information they gleaned, passed down through millennia, is extraordinarily valuable.

Fortunately, today there is a trend toward the fusion of modern psychology and ancient wisdom. Lewis Mehl-Madrona, MD, PhD, a Native American psychiatrist and author of the seminal book *Coyote Medicine,* spoke about "Indigenous Models of the Mind and Mental Health Care" at the 2010 integrative mental health conference in Phoenix. I invited him to be on our faculty to bring a very different perspective to the event. Dr. Mehl-Madrona says of the Lakota (Sioux) people, "The Lakota language does not have a concept of strictly mental health. Health is always seen as being part of one's entire being, of the community's entire being, existing in a state of balance and harmony." Each person is regarded as "an intimate part of the natural world, not separate from it," he says.

> In these ways of thinking of the mind and mental health, the *community* is the basic unit of study, not the individual.... The idea is that we are formed by our relationships. It is not that our brain makes our relationships, but rather our relationships make our brains.... Developmental neuroscientists are discovering that relationships actually physically structure our brains. Relationships with parents and care-givers actually create the brain.... We are relational selves. We are not individual, autonomous units. The elders think that's a ridiculous way of thinking. "How could you ever think such a thing?" they would say.

Mehl-Madrona told the story of a colleague who argued that the Lakota were "too primitive to benefit from psychotherapy." He responded, "It's not that we're primitive. It's just that we don't think it's very interesting to try to have a conversation with a person who sits behind us and won't talk back." He also stressed the importance of having a circle of friends to meet with regularly in order to support health and healing with directed energy, thoughts, and prayers. "How many of you have that kind of support?" he asked the audience of mental health professionals. "If you were sick—physically or emotionally—where would you find it?"

The Native American emphasis on community as a pillar of emotional well-being is an example of traditional wisdom usually neglected by today's mental health professions. Therapies based on community, like the sweat lodge, purification rituals, and prayer circles, might be useful to people suffering from depression or wanting to enjoy greater resilience, contentment, comfort, and serenity. Such approaches are integrative by nature, addressing all dimensions of human experience—physical, mental, social, and spiritual.

By *spiritual* I mean our nonmaterial essence, that aspect of our being that connects us to the essence of all other beings and to everything in the universe. Spirituality and religion share some common ground, but spirituality is not synonymous with religion. I consider it an important component of health and have made sure that Spirituality in Medicine is part of the integrative medicine curriculum at the University of Arizona. Chapter 7 discusses the role of secular spirituality in emotional well-being.

Of the spiritual traditions of the world, the one that has most to offer to the developing integrative model of mental health is Buddhism. Buddhism is a popular religion, with some 360 million adherents, mostly in Asia, and of course, like other religions, it has its share of dogma, ritual, and required belief in supernatural phenomena. But the founder of Buddhism was a philosopher, not a deity, a man who probed deeply into the nature of reality and the human mind and who devoted his life to understanding unhappiness and discontent and the possibility of alleviating them. One of his fundamental teachings was that life is *dukka,* a Sanskrit term usually translated as "suffering" but possibly better rendered as "incompleteness" or "unfulfillment." In any case, *dukka* is very far from contentment and happiness. He attributed this essential quality of our experience to our awareness of the impermanence of everything—nothing in our lives is immune to decay and death—as well as to the deeply rooted tendency of our minds to try to hold on to what is pleasant and shun what is unpleasant. And he taught specific practices to help people free themselves from suffering.

Although Buddhist philosophy predates the field of psychology by more than two thousand years, contemporary students of the mind are finding it a rich source of concepts and methods to improve emotional well-being. In recent years, Buddhist teachers from Tibet have been most active in bringing these ideas to the Western world. Tenzin Gyatso, the fourteenth Dalai Lama, who developed an active interest in science as a child, invited American lawyer and entrepreneur R. Adam Engle and Chilean biologist and neuroscientist Francisco J. Varela (1946–2001) to convene the first Mind and Life Dialogue in Dharamsala, India, in 1987; the intent was to foster collaboration between Buddhism and the cognitive sciences. Afterward the trio cofounded the Mind and Life Institute, a nonprofit organization affiliated with leading scientific researchers. The Dalai Lama is the honorary chairman and since its founding has participated in twenty-three of the Institute's annual dialogues. Mind and Life XV, held in 2007 at Emory University in Atlanta, was titled "Mindfulness, Compassion, and the Treatment of Depression." The experts in attendance—a mix of neuroscientists, psychologists, and Buddhist teachers—were invited to have a dialogue about "depression in physiological and cognitive terms so as to explore the possibility that mindfulness-based therapies, along with techniques to enhance compassion, may prove especially useful in the treatment of depression." They concurred that this was a promising direction for future research.

Neuroscientists have been prominent in this initiative from its beginning. As a result of their meetings with advanced Buddhist practitioners, some of them have begun to document differences in the brain associated with training in meditation and the development of compassion and empathy. The most significant finding of neuroscientific research influenced by Buddhist philosophy is that learning to change our ways of thinking and perceiving can actually change the function and structure of our brains. This is strong evidence for the deficiency of the biomedical model of mental health, which regards brain activity and biochemistry as primary. In the biomedical model, it is twisted molecules that cause twisted thoughts, never the other way around. As I explained in the previous chapter, the limited usefulness of that belief system is revealed in its limited ability to alleviate negative emotional states through psychopharmacological interventions. In the integrative model, the arrows of cause and effect point in both directions: from mind to brain as well as from brain to mind.

The leading researcher in this field is Richard Davidson, who directs the Laboratory for Affective Neuroscience as well as the Waisman Laboratory for Brain Imaging and Behavior, both at the University of Wisconsin–Madison. Davidson is bringing scientific rigor to the study of Buddhist practices and their ability to enhance emotional well-being by using advanced brain-imaging technologies, such as quantitative electrophysiology, positron emission tomography (PET), and functional magnetic resonance imaging (fMRI). He is particularly interested in the potential of meditation to alter brain function and structure over both the short and long term.

Davidson has focused on interactions between two areas of the brain, one modern and one ancient in evolutionary terms. The prefrontal cortex is the forwardmost part of the frontal lobes, believed to be responsible for complex reasoning and social behavior, while the almond-shaped amygdalae, located deep within the brain, are thought to mediate primal emotional responses, especially fear and rage. In other words, Davidson tracks how thoughts generated in the modern brain can modify reactions — and, eventually, structures — in the ancient brain.

Davidson's studies, along with those of others, demonstrate that neuroplasticity is a fundamental characteristic of our brains. Among other things, neuroplasticity means that emotions such as happiness and compassion can be cultivated in much the same way that a person can learn through repetition to play golf and basketball or master a musical instrument, and that such practice changes the activity and physical aspects of specific brain areas. In a reversal of the biomedical axiom, Davidson has shown that there are no peaceful molecules without peaceful thoughts.

One early subject of his studies was Matthieu Ricard, a French academic with a PhD in molecular genetics–turned–Buddhist monk. Ricard has been dubbed "The World's Happiest Man" because of his outstanding scores in tests performed in Davidson's lab. MRI scans of the brain show that he and other long-term meditators have vastly increased activity in the left prefrontal cortex, which is associated with positive emotional states, along with suppressed activity of the right prefrontal cortex, which is more active in those with mood disorders. Each of the meditators tested had completed more than ten thousand hours of meditation, and all showed this pattern of activity, but Ricard did so far more than others. In a January 2007 interview, Ricard told the British newspaper *The Independent* that "the mind is malleable." He said, "Our life can be greatly transformed by even a minimal change in how we manage our thoughts and perceive and interpret the world. Happiness is a skill. It requires effort and time."

The Dalai Lama, who believes that "the purpose of life is happiness," also teaches that "happiness can be achieved through training the mind." He says that happiness "is determined more by the state of one's mind than by one's external conditions, circumstances, or events— at least once one's basic survival needs are met." Together with psychiatrist Howard C. Cutler, MD, he has authored a classic manual on the subject: *The Art of Happiness: A Handbook for Living.* It is unlikely that many of us who are not Buddhist monks would be willing to invest ten thousand hours in the practice of meditation to master this art, but there are other, more time-efficient ways of doing so—for example, by cultivating mindfulness.

"Right mindfulness" is one of the main components of the Buddhist prescription for liberation from suffering. It is usually interpreted as calm awareness of one's body, mind, and content of consciousness. The concept has helped inspire the modern field of positive psychology and is prominent in numerous self-help books emphasizing it as the key to reducing stress and optimizing emotional well-being.* Psychologists think of mindfulness as the self-regulation of attention and the ability to maintain attention on one's experience in the present moment. Most of us are unconscious of the focus of our awareness. We let it drift to random thoughts, images in the "mind's eye," memories of the past, hopes and fears for the future. It takes motivation and practice to over-

---

* A good example and one that I recommend is *Log On: Two Steps to Mindful Awareness* by Amit Sood, MD (BookSurge, 2009).

come these natural tendencies and bring full attention to the present moment, and even more practice to be nonjudgmental about what comes into it. The goal is to acknowledge whatever comes—thoughts, images, sensations—and not label them as pleasant or unpleasant, not try to hold on to them or avoid them, not associate them with painful past memories or future desires.

Mindfulness training as a psychological tool is now widely used in a variety of settings, from hospitals to corporate offices. For example, many health professionals make use of mindfulness-based stress reduction (MBSR) to help patients cope with chronic pain and disease. MBSR, which includes yoga, focused breathing, and basic meditation, can be learned quickly by anyone. Studies show it to be effective at improving outcomes and quality of life in patients with chronic pain and a variety of diseases, such as rheumatoid arthritis, cancer, and HIV. And MBSR may change brain structure and function quickly. In a study reported in January 2011 in *Psychiatry Research: Neuroimaging,* a team of American and German researchers described MRIs from sixteen healthy participants before and after they underwent an eight-week MBSR program. Compared to those of the controls, the brains of those who completed MBSR training showed increases in the posterior cingulate cortex, the temporoparietal junction, and the cerebellum. The researchers' conclusion: "The results suggest that participation in MBSR is associated with changes in gray matter concentration in brain regions involved in learning and memory processes, emotion regulation, self-referential processing, and perspective taking."

Another application, mindfulness-based cognitive therapy (MBCT), incorporates information about depression and strategies to increase awareness of the link between thoughts and feelings. Through MBCT, those who are prone to depression can learn to recognize patterns of thinking associated with negative moods and change them.

Daniel Siegel, MD, clinical professor of psychiatry at UCLA, where he also codirects the Mindful Awareness Research Center, calls this ability "mindsight":

Mindsight is a kind of focused attention that allows us to see the internal workings of our own minds. It helps us to be aware of our mental processes without being swept away by them, enables us to get ourselves off the autopilot of imagined behaviors and habitual responses, and moves us beyond the reactive emotional loops we all have a tendency to get trapped in. It lets us "name and tame" the emotions we are experiencing rather than be overwhelmed by them.

Consider the difference between speaking and thinking, "I **am** sad" and "I **feel** sad." Similar as those two statements may seem, there is actually a profound difference between them. "I am sad" is a kind of self-definition and a very limiting one. "I feel sad" suggests the ability to recognize and acknowledge a feeling without being consumed by it. The focusing skills that are a part of mindsight make it possible to distinguish between the feeling and the identity, accept the present moment of that feeling, let it go, and then transform it.

We now know from the findings of neuroscience research that the mental and emotional changes we can create through cultivation of the skill of mindsight are transformational at the very physical level of the brain. By developing the ability to focus our attention on our internal world, we pick up a "scalpel" we can use to resculpt our neural pathways, stimulating the growth of areas that are crucial to mental health.... This revelation is based on one of the most exciting scientific discoveries of the last twenty years: How we focus our attention shapes the structure of the brain. Neuroscience supports the idea that developing the reflective skills of mindsight activates the very circuits that create resilience and well-being and that underlie empathy and compassion as well.

I first became interested in learning to focus my attention as a result of reading about Zen Buddhism in my late twenties. On my own, I began to sit each morning and try to keep my attention on my breath, counting each outbreath from one to ten, then starting over from one on the inbreath. Most of the time, I would find myself up to twenty- or thirty-something without even being aware of going past ten, my attention having wandered to thoughts or images in my mind. The difficulty of what seemed like an easy task surprised me and made me aware for the first time in my life of the restless nature of the mind. I took it as a challenge and kept at it.

Later I took formal training in *vipassana,* also known as "insight meditation," a tradition from Southeast Asian Buddhism introduced to the West more recently. Its purpose is to develop insight into the nature of consciousness through mindsight, creating nonjudgmental openness to body sensations, thoughts, and feelings, noting them and letting them pass. Again, I found this very challenging.

I still find it difficult. Even after forty years of practice I have made minimal progress at curbing my mental restlessness. But I sensed that meditation was valuable for me long before there was any neuroscientific research on its beneficial effects. I don't feel quite right if I miss a period—however brief—of sitting still and focusing my attention at the start of a day, and I believe this practice is one reason that my episodes of dysthymia have diminished in both frequency and severity. Learning to focus attention has also helped me work more efficiently.

Sitting meditation is not the only way to develop this skill. For example, cooking for me is a form of meditation. When I chop vegetables, I am fully in the moment. If I weren't, I would be more likely to cut myself with the sharp knives I use and not get the pieces just as I want them. Preparing a meal from fresh ingredients requires juggling many variables in order to have all the dishes come out exactly right at the same time. It also is an exercise in manifestation: bringing the idea of a dish first into the visual imagination, then into reality—most fun when I don't follow a recipe. Public speaking gives me another opportunity to be highly focused. I speak without notes and cannot allow my attention to wander when I do so. My preferred physical activity in recent years has been swimming. When I swim, I naturally concentrate on my breathing.

Overcoming depression and creating emotional well-being by cultivating mindfulness and focused attention and becoming aware of and managing the interactions between thoughts and feelings are examples of psychological tools based on ancient wisdom. I consider them essential components of an integrative approach to mental health and will give you specific recommendations for using them in chapter 6. They are even more powerful when combined with lifestyle changes that address other factors that undermine our emotional resilience.

I have reviewed a few lifestyle programs intended to relieve depression by correcting the mismatch between the modern world and our "ancient brains and bodies." They recommend such interventions as increasing aerobic exercise, improving sleep, spending more time in the sun, eating more fish to boost intake of omega-3 fatty acids, socializing more, and not dwelling on negative thoughts.*

This is a good start, but I consider the program I present in this book much more comprehensive. It integrates many more effective recommendations based on the latest scientific evidence. Replicating the hunter-gatherer lifestyle of our distant ancestors has merit, but I am not persuaded that it is the whole answer. Structured meditation and cultivation of mindsight did not exist in the hunter-gatherer world, for example, but, as I have explained, neuroscientists are demonstrating that they can change our brains for the better and improve our moods. And they may be useful tools to help people disengage from negative thoughts—never an easy task.

The recommendations I give you in part 2 of this book have a larger purpose than managing depression. They are designed to increase your emotional resilience, allow you to move your emotional set point toward more positive moods, and give you greater opportunity to enjoy the resilience, contentment, comfort, and serenity that characterize emotional well-being. By doing so, you will increase your chances of experiencing spontaneous happiness more often, the kind of happiness that comes from within and is always available because it does not depend on external circumstances or the vagaries of fortune.

---

* See, for example, Stephen Ilardi's *The Depression Cure.*

PART TWO

PRACTICE

5

Optimizing Emotional Well-Being by Caring for the Body

Physical Disease and Emotions

It should come as no surprise that physical and emotional health are intertwined and impossible to tease apart. From the perspective of integrative medicine, mind and body are two aspects of an underlying unity, so that changes in one always correlate with changes in the other. Of course, conventional biology-explains-all medicine has long recognized anxiety, depression, and other disturbances of mood as symptoms of physical disease, but it has been slow to accept the possibility that imbalances in the mental/emotional realm can cause physical symptoms. I am happy to see that change as new research illuminates the complex interactions of mind and body. The findings also suggest powerful strategies for improving emotional well-being through physical interventions.

Textbooks I used in medical school included mood disturbances among symptoms of endocrine disorders, which are conditions that involve hormone-secreting glands such as the thyroid, adrenals, and pituitary. A classic example is the association of depression with hypothyroidism. Up to 20 percent of people suffering from depression are deficient in thyroid hormones; many of them have received long-term treatment with antidepressant drugs before physicians thought to check their thyroid function. That should be assessed in every depressed patient and, if low, corrected. Thyroid hormones regulate metabolism; just how they affect our emotions is not known. They may have direct effects on brain centers or may influence the production and recycling of neurotransmitters. Dysfunction of the pituitary and adrenal glands also commonly affects emotional health, as do the drugs used to treat it. In Addison's disease, for example, the immune system damages the adrenal cortex and its ability to produce cortisol and other vitally important hormones; irritability and depression are common symptoms, along with many physical changes. The corticosteroid drugs required to keep patients with Addison's disease alive and healthy can cause both mania and depression.*

It is well known that sex hormones affect mood in both men and women. Emotional changes associated with the female menstrual cycle and with menopause are often striking. Depression in some older men can be relieved by boosting low testosterone levels. Presumably, sex hormones have direct effects on the brain and on neurotransmitters involved with our emotions. More curious is the influence of insulin, the hormone secreted by the pancreas that controls blood sugar (glucose) and the production and distribution of energy in the body. People with diabetes are more likely to be depressed than people without it. Some studies link depression to insulin resistance, the underlying problem in the more common type-2 variety of diabetes, but we don't know what is cause and what is effect. Insulin receptors occur throughout the brain. Might this hormone directly affect mood? A recent study in animals with type-1 diabetes demonstrated a previously unknown effect of insulin on dopamine signaling in key brain centers. Or is it that the dis-

---

* Concern about this possibility in one Addison's sufferer, John F. Kennedy (1917–1963), the thirty-fifth president of the United States, led his doctors and managers to conceal the diagnosis and treatment from the public.

turbed glucose metabolism of diabetes alters brain function? (Brain cells rely on glucose as their sole source of energy and must have a constant supply of it.) Or is the source of diabetics' depression the fact that they have a serious chronic disease that can undermine quality of life?

We might also ask that about the occurrence of depression in conjunction with other serious chronic diseases that are not rooted in hormonal imbalances. One in three heart attack survivors experiences depression, as does one in four people who have strokes and one in three patients with HIV. Certainly, such patients have reason to be depressed, but how much of their depression might be a symptom of their disease rather than a psychological reaction to it?

We have no evidence that HIV directly affects emotions, but cardiovascular disease, even before it progresses to heart attacks and strokes, often impairs blood flow to the brain, and this might disturb the function of centers that control emotions. An even higher percentage—50 percent—of people with Parkinson's disease suffer from depression. Here, altered brain biochemistry is the likely explanation, because this progressive condition causes degeneration of neurons that use dopamine to signal other neurons in the midbrain, specifically in centers controlling movement but also in other parts of the brain, including the frontal lobes. It may damage serotonin pathways as well. One research neurologist who has studied the correlation of depression and Parkinson's, Irene Richards, MD, of the University of Rochester (New York) Medical Center, says unequivocally, "The depression is part of the illness, not simply a reaction to the disease."

The obvious takeaway message from this is to make sure that a physical problem is not responsible for suboptimal emotional wellness, especially an easily treatable one like hypothyroidism. So, one of my first recommendations in the list at the end of this chapter is to get a complete medical checkup, including necessary blood tests, if you have not had one recently. A more subtle conclusion I draw is that inquiry into the mechanisms linking disease and emotions can provide valuable information that we all would do well to make use of in adjusting our ways of living. I base that conclusion on my reading of the scientific literature on the common association of depression with another serious chronic disease that we are all familiar with: cancer.

DEPRESSION AND INFLAMMATION: THE CYTOKINE CONNECTION

As many as 25 percent of persons with cancer experience depression. With some kinds of cancer—notably pancreatic—the percentage is much higher. In some cases depression precedes the diagnosis of cancer; in others it comes afterward. Medical scientists speculate endlessly about possible explanations for the association of these conditions. Some think that depression might be an early symptom of a pancreatic tumor, especially in men. Others think the relationship is more likely to be indirect. Maybe smoking is the hidden link: cigarette smoking is a known risk factor for pancreatic cancer, and tobacco addiction is more common in people prone to emotional problems. Or chemotherapy might be to blame for the depression. Often, it has profound mental and emotional side effects: irritability and impairment of memory and concentration as well as mood. (*Chemo brain* is the common term for these symptoms; fortunately, they usually dissipate sometime after treatment ends.)

Recently another hypothesis—and, to my mind, a very compelling one—has attracted attention. Based on animal research models, it proposes a mechanism that links the brain and the immune system to explain cancer-related symptoms, including emotional changes. I believe it offers new possibilities for preventing and treating depression and enhancing emotional well-being. The mechanism centers on cytokines, potent regulatory proteins made by immune cells that govern responses to foreign antigens and germs. People with cancer often have abnormal immunity due to abnormal production and function of cytokines.

Cytokines have diverse effects. One type—the interleukins—controls inflammation and produces fever. Another type governs the maturation of red and white blood cells in the bone marrow. Yet another—the interferons—helps us defend against bacteria, parasites, viruses, and malignant cells; they are named for their ability to interfere with viral replication. A group of cytokines called tumor necrosis factors got their name because they can kill some cancer cells in test tubes; they regulate programmed cell suicide and general inflammation and are a significant part of the body's defensive reaction to the presence of malignant growth.

Some cytokines have proved useful as medical treatments despite significant toxicity. In 1980, scientists succeeded in inserting a gene for human interferon into bacteria, allowing mass production and purification. Since then, synthetic injectable forms of interferon have been in wide use as treatments for a number of kinds of cancer (skin cancers, some leukemias), chronic viral hepatitis, and multiple sclerosis. A commonly reported side effect of interferon therapy is severe depression; some patients have even killed themselves. One form of interleukin is used to treat metastatic kidney cancer and advanced melanoma. In addition to severe physical side effects, it can cause paranoia and hallucinations.

Long-term activation of the immune system, as in autoimmune disease, seems to go along with depression, and depression seems to involve changes in various aspects of immunity, particularly those having to do with cytokines. People with rheumatoid arthritis, scleroderma, systemic lupus erythematosus (SLE), and other forms of autoimmunity are often depressed. And when proinflammatory cytokines are administered to animals, they elicit "sickness behavior," a distinctive pattern of behavioral changes. The animals become listless, lose interest in eating, grooming, socializing, and sex, and show increased sensitivity to pain.

Farmers have long recognized this pattern in sick animals and attributed it to physical weakness, but in the 1960s, research revealed a blood-borne factor to be responsible. (Injections of blood from sick animals caused sickness behavior in healthy ones.) Believed to act on the brain, it was named factor X until the 1980s, when it was identified as proinflammatory cytokines made by activated white blood cells in response to bacterial antigens. Sickness behavior is an adaptive response of the organism that conserves energy and favors healing. It is also strikingly similar to the changes in behavior accompanying major depression—so similar, in fact, that researchers in the field of psycho-neuroimmunology have developed a cytokine hypothesis of depression, which argues that proinflammatory cytokines are the key factor controlling the behavioral, hormonal, and neurochemical alterations characteristic of depressive disorders, including much of the depression that occurs with cancer.

Loss of interest in food and a lack of pleasure in eating make sense as short-term responses to infection—they free up energy used for digestion and make it available for immune defense. Once the immune system gains the upper hand, it can turn down the cytokines, allowing brain centers that control appetite and taste to resume normal activity. Malignant tumors, however, even when they are relatively small, often stimulate prolonged cytokine responses that do more harm than good. For example, they are responsible for the permanent suppression of appetite and aversion to food that result in the extreme wasting (cachexia) that all too many cancer patients suffer. Given that dramatic effect on the brain and body, consider the impact of prolonged cytokine responses on parts of the brain associated with thoughts and emotions.

THE IMPORTANCE OF AN ANTI-INFLAMMATORY DIET AND LIFESTYLE

The reason I find the cytokine hypothesis of depression so compelling is that it fits right in with my belief that doing everything we can to contain unnecessary inflammation—by adhering to an anti-inflammatory diet, for example—is the best overall strategy for attaining optimum health and experiencing healthy aging. Let me briefly summarize this view.

Inflammation is the cornerstone of the body's healing response. It is the process by which the immune system delivers more nourishment and more defensive activity to an area that is injured or under attack. But inflammation is so powerful and so potentially destructive that it must stay where it is supposed to be and end when it is supposed to end; otherwise it damages the body and causes disease. We all know inflammation when it occurs on the surface of the body as local redness, heat, swelling, and pain; we are less aware of it when it affects us internally, particularly if it is chronic, diffuse, and low level. But chronic, diffuse, low-level inflammation inside the body—in the lining of arteries, in the brain, and in various other tissues and organs—is the root cause of the most common and serious diseases of aging, including cardiovascular disease, Alzheimer's (and other degenerative diseases of the central nervous system), and cancer. The link with cancer may seem less obvious, but it is quite real, because anything that promotes inflammation also promotes cell proliferation, increasing risks of malignant transformation. Cytokines are the principal chemical mediators of the inflammatory response. Anything you can do to keep them within their proper bounds will reduce your risks of chronic disease and also, it now appears, help protect you from depression.

Dietary choices are of great importance. In chapter 2 I pointed to modern industrial food as a possible cause of epidemic depression. We all know that fast food and junk food and the highly processed stuff that fills the shelves of supermarkets and convenience stores are not good for us. Now there is a powerful evidence-based argument for not eating this way: these new kinds of manufactured food promote inflammation. They are a principal reason why so many North Americans and people in other developed countries go through life in proinflammatory states with their cytokine systems in high gear. Industrial food fails to provide our bodies with protective nutrients (vitamins, minerals, and the phytonutrients—plant-derived compounds—most abundant in vegetables and fruits). At the same time, it gives us too many proinflammatory fats and carbohydrates.

The natural pigments that color vegetables and fruits; antioxidants in olive oil, tea, and chocolate; novel compounds in ginger, turmeric, and other spices and herbs; and the special fats in oily fish, all protect our tissues and organs from inappropriate inflammation; some are potent natural anti-inflammatory agents. Today's mainstream diet is glaringly deficient in these protective elements.

At the same time, it is overloaded with fats that promote inflammation: polyunsaturated vegetable oils (especially refined soybean oil, cheap and ubiquitous in industrial food products); margarine and other partially hydrogenated and trans fats; and fats in the meat of cows and chickens raised on unnatural grain-rich diets. All of these increase the production and activity of proinflammatory cytokines. And it gives us carbohydrates mostly in the form of products made from quick-digesting flour and sugar: bread, pastry, cookies, crackers, chips, sugary drinks, etc. These are classified as high-glycemic-load foods because they raise blood sugar quickly,* stimulate insulin resistance in the many of us who are genetically at risk for it, and increase inflammation, perhaps in several ways. Insulin resistance is associated with inflammation (and, as mentioned above, with depression). Also, the spikes of blood sugar that follow high-glycemic-load meals cause abnormal reactions between sugar and proteins throughout the body that produce proinflammatory compounds.** In the past, people ate mostly low-glycemic-load carbohydrate foods that digested slowly and did not cause blood sugar to spike, foods such as whole or cracked (as opposed to pulverized) grains, starchy roots and tubers, beans, and winter squashes.

I have designed an anti-inflammatory diet using the Mediterranean diet as a template. It is the way I eat and the way I recommend others eat to maintain optimum health. Based on my reading of the scientific literature on the relationship between inflammation and depression, I

---

* *Glycemia* is the medical term for sugar in the blood.
** The reactions are known as glycation reactions; the proinflammatory compounds they produce are advanced glycation end products (AGEs).

now recommend it to you as an effective strategy for attaining optimum emotional well-being, and I have included details of it in the program at the end of this book. I assure you that it is not hard to eat this way and that doing so does not in any way diminish the pleasure of eating. The most important rule is simply to avoid refined, processed, and manufactured foods. By taking that one step toward better nutrition, you can significantly reduce the proinflammatory pressures of modern living.

Keep in mind, however, that while diet may be the keystone of an anti-inflammatory lifestyle, it is not the only component. Many common environmental toxins and irritants trigger inflammation, among them tobacco smoke and other pollutants in air, water, and food, as well as chemicals in household products. It is a good idea to take sensible measures to limit exposure to them as well as increase your body's resistance to their effects—by using dietary supplements appropriately, for example. Exercise is also an important factor. People who are fit and who exercise regularly have less inflammation than others. That may be one reason physical activity has such a dramatic and beneficial effect on emotional well-being. (Many other mechanisms are also probably involved; I will review them in a moment.) The quantity and quality of your sleep also influence inflammation, as does stress. Crafting an effective anti-inflammatory lifestyle means attending to all of these factors.

Here are two case examples of dramatic mood improvement brought about by changing dietary habits.* Cham from Baltimore, Maryland, reports:

> Years ago every morning I would cry for about three hours. I couldn't even get out of bed. This had about 70 percent to do with the choices I was being pressured to make and 30 percent to do with the way I was handling my food intake. Counseling helped with the bad personal choices and removing the negative people in my

---

* These and many of the other personal stories in this book were solicited from readers of my website, www.drweil.com, and from my social media pages.

life, but it took me years to identify the nutrition challenge. I found that a generous helping of lean protein foods in the morning and avoidance of simple carbohydrates like sugar and refined wheat products had a dramatic effect on my mood. My breakfast now looks more like dinner, it may have lean meat, egg whites, tofu, beans, whole grains, yogurt, and always several vegetables. This works for me and would probably work for others as well. I'm no doctor, but I have been adjusting this nutrition plan for years, and I am confident that eating the right foods in the morning can help deter a morning plunge into depression.

Cham's story conforms to my personal experience. Typical American breakfast foods may be the worst possible choices for starting the day. Cereal, waffles, pancakes, muffins, toast with jam, cinnamon rolls, orange juice, and similar blood-sugar spikers virtually guarantee a crash in mood and energy by midmorning. When I first had a traditional Japanese breakfast of fish, vegetables, miso soup, and a modest portion of steamed rice, it was an utter revelation. I now always eat protein — especially fish or whole soy — with breakfast and try to avoid high-glycemic-load carbohydrates.

Carol, from Finleyville, Pennsylvania, also has learned the importance of a dietary makeover to create a new mind and mood:

> In 2003, I was overweight. I was a confirmed "bakery-o-holic," "Dorito- and Pepsi-o-holic," and was living on ibuprofen and quite a few other prescription drugs....I made up my mind it was all the crap that I was eating that was making me horribly depressed and overweight. Not only did I need knee replacements, I had fibromyalgia — I was a physical and mental mess.
>
> So between 2003 and 2005, I taught myself a whole new lifestyle....I would like to take the opportunity to THANK YOU from the bottom of my heart, because you were the one that taught me to eat right, take the right supplements. To this day I only take an occasional ibuprofen, if all else fails.

Here I am at almost age sixty-four, and happy as can be with my fifty-pound weight loss over the course of seven years, and LOVING exercise and eating and cooking. I just can't believe the difference in my mental well-being now compared to how I felt in 2003. I cook vegetarian, and eat WILD seafood only. I try to eat organic when I can....

My observation is that my mental well-being is linked to the right food and the right supplements, and exercise!

DIETARY SUPPLEMENTS AND EMOTIONAL WELL-BEING

Many studies link specific nutrient deficiencies to suboptimal brain function and mental/emotional health. The most important by far is lack of omega-3 fatty acids. These special fats are critically important for both physical and mental health. The body needs regular daily intake of adequate amounts of both EPA and DHA, two long-chain omega-3 fats that are abundant in oily fish from cold northern waters but otherwise are hard to come by. Most of us do not get enough, making this the most serious dietary deficiency in our population. A great deal of scientific data links low tissue levels of EPA and DHA to a host of mental/emotional disorders, including depression, violent behavior, suicide, and learning disabilities. Dietary supplementation with these fats, usually in the form of fish oil, has proved to be an effective, natural, and nontoxic therapy for bipolar disorder, attention deficit hyperactivity disorder, postpartum depression, seasonal affective disorder, and more. It also helps prevent depression and improve overall emotional well-being. Very high doses of fish oil — 20 grams a day or more — have been used as treatments without any ill effects. In fact, there is no downside to adding fish oil to your diet (except for the sustainability of ocean resources, a significant concern).

Human beings are literally fatheads — fat accounts for about 60 percent of the dry weight of our brains. Omega-3 fatty acids optimize brain health in several ways. DHA is the main structural component of nerve cell membranes; if it is deficient in the diet, especially during embryonic development, infancy, and early childhood, brain "architecture" will be weak, leaving the central nervous system more vulnerable to harmful effects of stress and environmental toxins and impairing its function. Both EPA and DHA reduce inflammation, and both protect neurons from injury and improve communication between them. They also contribute to the health of the cardiovascular system and its ability to meet the brain's need for uninterrupted supplies of oxygen and glucose.

The human need for abundant omega-3s is explained by our evolutionary history. Many anthropologists now believe that humans broke away from the primate pack and developed large, complex brains when they figured out how to secure animal foods rich in omega-3 fatty acids, especially fish. A gorilla, eating mostly leaves and other raw vegetable matter that is very low in fats, has a brain that is about 0.2 percent of overall body weight, while a human's brain is 3 percent of body weight; in relative terms, that's *15 times larger*.

The anti-inflammatory diet emphasizes omega-3-rich fish as a main source of animal protein, especially sockeye salmon, black cod, sardines, and herring, all "good" species with regard to both sustainability and toxic contamination (with mercury, PCBs, etc.). I eat these fish often and also take 3 grams of supplemental fish oil a day. Because an omega-3 deficiency is so common, and raising tissue levels of omega-3s has so many health benefits in general, I recommend that everyone take 2 to 4 grams of a good fish oil product every day. (I give product specifications on page 204.) I cannot overemphasize the importance of this simple measure to improve emotional well-being. Not only does it offer real protection against depression, but I believe it can help move your emotional set point away from sadness and toward contentment. Of all the body-oriented interventions I discuss in this chapter, the two that I prescribe most frequently are regular physical activity (see page 89) and supplemental fish oil.

Margo, forty-nine, an engineer and wellness consultant from Pottstown, Pennsylvania, uses fish oil to reduce her dependence on pharmaceuticals:

> There is a long history of depression and alcoholism on both sides of my family, including my immediate family. After finally admitting that I, too, had a problem with depression, I went on antidepressants. For years I was fine. Then, slowly, I weaned myself off one of the two drugs and within six months I reached a new depth of despair, which was then relieved by going back on the second medication. I now am doing very well on minimal dosage of each since I added omega-3 to my daily diet. I am taking the most potent supplement available. I feel better than I remember feeling for a long time and plan to stay on omega-3 for life and get off drugs, if I can.

Pregnant women are particularly vulnerable to depleted omega-3 fatty acid stores. If dietary sources are inadequate, the fetus will rob the mother's tissues of the omega-3s it needs for brain and nervous system development, leaving her at high risk for pre- and postpartum depression. Kari, thirty, a clinical social worker from Antioch, California, tells this story:

> When I was in my seventh month of my first pregnancy, my hormones left me feeling so overwhelmed. Anything could trigger my heart pounding and teary eyes to well. I had taken my usual vitamin regimen, but adding fish oil helped keep my negative emotions at bay. I felt normal again and noticed that if I missed a day, my anxiety and tearfulness would creep back in.

Carol, sixty, a finance-industry manager from Lake Dallas, Texas, says she suffered from depression and posttraumatic stress disorder for "most of my adult life" but attributes a turnaround principally to two sources of omega-3 fats—fish oil and walnuts:

After about three weeks of daily use I find that my flat mood and malaise have been replaced by a lighter and more upbeat feeling. The change is subtle but real. I highly recommend this as a trial for anyone who prefers to not use antidepressants (the serotonin reuptake inhibitors always made me sleepy—way too sleepy—like all day long). Actually I tried Prozac and Paxil in the 1980s and couldn't tell a benefit at all, so I would say that for my particular chemistry and issues, fish oil and walnuts trumped drugs.

Walnuts and other vegetarian sources of omega-3s, such as chia seeds and the seeds and oils of flax and hemp, do not provide EPA and DHA. They provide only a short-chain precursor (ALA) that the body must convert to the long-chain compounds it needs. That conversion is inefficient at best and is further inhibited in the presence of the fats that predominate in processed food. Flax and hemp seeds and walnuts are good additions to the diet, but they are not substitutes for fish and fish oil.

I am conflicted about telling people to eat more fish and take fish oil, because overfishing has so depleted the world's oceans. I am involved with ongoing efforts to develop a sustainable source of omega-3s from algae. Salmon and other oily fish do not make their own EPA and DHA; no animal can do that. Instead, they get them by eating the algae that do make their own. A commercial algae-derived DHA product is now available, but it is hard to find one containing both EPA and DHA. Soon, I hope, I will be able to use and advise others to use an algae-derived omega-3 supplement that is equivalent to fish oil, one suitable for vegetarians and for all of us who care about the state of our oceans.

The second most common and serious nutritional deficiency in our population is lack of vitamin D, actually a hormone made in the skin on exposure to ultraviolet light from the sun. For various reasons, many people do not get adequate sun exposure to meet their needs for vitamin D, and it is almost impossible to get enough of it from diet alone. Supplementation, however, is effective and inexpensive. A recent explosion of research on vitamin D has made both doctors and laypeople aware of its myriad benefits, not just for bone health but for protection against many kinds of cancer, multiple sclerosis, influenza, and other diseases. As a result, more doctors now routinely check blood levels of vitamin D in their patients and are documenting a deficiency in many of them.

Less well known are the connections between vitamin D, brain health, and emotional well-being. Receptors for vitamin D occur throughout the brain, and it appears to play an important role in the development and function of that organ, including the activity of neurotransmitters that affect mood. High vitamin D levels may protect against age-related cognitive decline. Low levels are associated with impaired cognitive function (especially in the elderly), seasonal affective disorder, depression, and even psychosis. (The last correlation is posed as a possible explanation for the surprisingly high incidence of schizophrenia in dark-skinned immigrants who move to northern European countries; dark-skinned people already have difficulty making enough vitamin D.)

As with omega-3 fatty acids, the benefits of vitamin D on both physical and mental health are so numerous and the deficiency so common that it is wise to supplement the diet with it. I take at least 2,000 IU a day and tell others to do that as well. Unlike with omega-3s, excessive intake of vitamin D can cause problems (too much calcium in the blood and tissues and possible kidney damage), but that happens only if doses far in excess of 2,000 IU a day are taken over time. There is no risk of vitamin D overdose from sun exposure, which has direct benefits on mood independent of its role in vitamin D synthesis. I will explain those benefits later in this chapter and tell you how to get them safely, without increasing the risk of skin cancer.

Below is a personal story of the power this micronutrient can exert over mood, from Christine, who lives in Beaverton, Oregon. While her intake is above my recommendation, research has found no adverse effects with supplemental vitamin D below 10,000 IU daily, so she is probably safe at this level. Indeed, in this cloudy, rainy, relatively northerly part of the country, she might be right on target:

I have found that taking a liquid vitamin D supplement has drastically improved my mood. While pregnant with my first child in 2007, I started taking 4,000 IU of vitamin D daily. After his birth, I increased it to 6,000 IU. I am currently pregnant again and am down to 4,000 IU, but, as someone who has struggled with mild to moderate depression her whole life, I have noticed that this has really been the one thing that has had a positive impact on my mood.

And here's a report from Christina, another northerner, who lives in Springfield, Massachusetts:

I am amazed at how much vitamin D has changed my life. I am taking a daily supplement now after a blood test showed me to be deficient. My nurse practitioner put me on a vitamin D regimen, and I soon felt so much calmer and more energetic. And I sleep better. If I forget to take it for a couple of days, I notice the depression seeping back in again.

Deficiencies of other vitamins and trace minerals have been reported in people with mood disorders. Correcting the deficiencies with dietary supplements sometimes helps. Most frequently cited is the B-complex of vitamins, a group of water-soluble compounds that the body cannot store and needs constantly for optimum metabolism. Its need for them is increased by stress, erratic diets, use of drugs and alcohol, smoking, illness, shift work, and demanding travel. Vitamins B-6, B-12, and folate are commonly included in over-the-counter formulas for depression; data are best for the first two, less solid for folate. There is no reason not to take the whole complex of B-vitamins in supplement form, but also no reason to take them separately from a daily multivitamin/multimineral supplement.

Micronutrient deficiencies are common in our population. Industrial food often provides suboptimal amounts, and many poor people cannot afford the fruits and vegetables that are the best sources. I have argued that giving all school kids a free multivitamin/multimineral supplement would be a cost-effective public health measure, one that I believe would improve performance and behavior in classrooms as well as the health of our young people. I am also on record as saying that dietary supplements are not substitutes for good diets. At best, they are partial representations of the full spectrum of protective elements in whole foods. But they are good insurance against gaps in the diet and may, as in the case of vitamin D, offer specific therapeutic and preventive benefits that cannot be obtained from diet alone. I grow a lot of my own food, prepare it myself, and am thoughtful about what I eat. I also take a good daily multivitamin/multimineral supplement and advise you to do so, too, because I consider it another safe and effective measure to optimize emotional well-being. The program in this book tells you how to identify the best products.

THE CRITICAL IMPORTANCE OF PHYSICAL ACTIVITY

A national news story from June 2010 described an "unorthodox treatment for anxiety and mood disorders, including depression" that was "free and has no side effects." The treatment was "nothing more than exercise."

Human bodies are designed for regular physical activity; the inactivity characteristic of so many people today undermines both general health and brain health and probably plays a significant role in the epidemic incidence of depression today. It is one of the most significant differences between the lifestyles of "advanced" societies and those of primitive ones, like the hunter-gatherers I mentioned in chapter 2, who enjoy much greater contentment than we do and among whom major depression is virtually unknown. More than two thousand years ago, the classical Greek philosopher Plato wrote: "In order for man to succeed in life, god provided him with two means, education and physical activity. Not separately, one for the soul and the other for the body, but for the two together. With these two means, men can attain perfection."

Many studies show that depressed patients who stick to a regimen of aerobic exercise improve as much as those treated with medication and are less likely to relapse. The data also suggest that exercise prevents depression and boosts mood in healthy people. More research is needed to reveal how exercise does this and to determine just how much and what kind works best, but given what we now know, I consider it inexcusable to omit exercise from an integrative treatment plan for emotional well-being. If the mainstream mental health professions do not yet endorse this prescription, it can only be explained by how little emphasis is placed on exercise in professional training and how little attention it gets in professional media. That and the fact that medical scientists say that research to date is methodologically weak.

The problem is that most of the studies on exercise and mood are cross-sectional in nature, meaning that they look at groups of people in one moment of time and observe correlations, such as better moods with regular physical activity. Studies of that kind are relatively easy to do and cost relatively little, but they do not allow us to draw solid cause-and-effect conclusions. Maybe people who are more physically active are more likely to behave in other ways that make them happier, or maybe genetic traits that make people more active also influence brain activity in ways that favor positive moods. If so, prescribing exercise to improve emotional well-being might not be effective as a general measure. What we need more of are longitudinal or prospective studies that follow groups of people over time and assess their moods as they stick to exercise regimens. Results of the few such studies that have been done generally support the effectiveness of regular exercise to maintain and enhance emotional wellness.

Many possible mechanisms are proposed for this effect, both neurobiological and psychological. There is no consensus, and my guess is that no one mechanism is responsible. We don't need to know how exercise works to improve our moods, but we do want to know how best to take advantage of it. Most prospective studies have used walking or jogging programs, but some research finds nonaerobic exercise such as strength and flexibility training as well as yoga to be effective, too. In *Yoga for Emotional Balance,* clinical psychologist and yoga therapist Bo Forbes explains:

> Posture and movement can be insidious in building anxiety and depression. Without realizing it, we repeat physical patterns hundreds of times daily, sharpening them on the whetstone of our experience.... Depression can imprint not only your movement patterns, but your posture as well. Your body may have what I call "Closed Heart Syndrome," a postural pattern that illustrates the helplessness, hopelessness, and self-protective withdrawal of depression. In Closed Heart Syndrome, the chest sinks and the heart area collapses. This makes the breath shallow and slow. The upper spine and shoulders round, as though to protect the heart from further disappointment. This also protects us from intimacy, which people with depression may see as merely another chance to be hurt....We use head and neck alignment, heart-opening restorative postures, and deep breathing to lift and balance depression. People who have physical symptoms of depression often benefit from lengthening and opening the upper thoracic spine and chest areas.

Typical therapeutic exercise programs last for eight to fourteen weeks with three to four sessions a week of at least twenty to thirty minutes. For treatment of depression and anxiety disorders, activities of moderate intensity, like brisk walking, are more successful than vigorous activity. The most important conclusions of research to date are that regular physical activity:

- is as effective a treatment for mild to moderate depression as antidepressant medication
- is an effective treatment for anxiety disorders
- in healthy people helps prevent both depression and anxiety

Increasing my own physical activity is one of the main measures that have helped me keep my dysthymia in check, but the kinds of activity I have used over the years have changed. In my thirties and early forties, I ran three miles or so most days of the week, until I began to notice that my knees did not like it. I phased out running and spent more time hiking and cycling. Later, I came to rely on exercise machines — stationary bikes, stair climbers, and elliptical trainers — as well as workouts with weights, both on my own and under the direction of a personal trainer. I also did some yoga for stretching and better balance. By the time I turned sixty, I came to regard such workouts as drudgery, too boring to keep me motivated. I started swimming regularly. My older body likes swimming very much, and I find that concentrating on my breathing as I swim is both meditative and relaxing. I try to swim most days. I also go on walks with my dogs and with friends and work in my garden. My colleague Victoria Maizes, MD, executive director of the Arizona Center for Integrative Medicine, tells her patients that they need exercise only on days that they eat. I agree that the goal is to get some physical activity every day.

More and more, I have come to believe that integrative exercise offers more health benefits, both physical and emotional, than other sorts. *Integrative exercise* means exercise necessary to accomplish some task. It is what our bodies are designed for — the activities of daily living. It is what people in premodern societies do. They walk, often uphill and downhill and over uneven ground, climb, lift, carry loads, chop wood, and so forth. The healthy and happy old people I've met in Okinawa and other parts of the world are regularly active in these ways; none of them use exercise machines, attend aerobics classes, or work with personal trainers. Research suggests that integrative exercise conditions our bodies most effectively, and that people are more inclined to stick with this kind of exercise. I believe that a major reason people abandon workout regimes based on treadmills, weight lifting, and other gym-based exercise is that, deep in our primitive psyches, we feel that such activity wastes energy. That feeling may be in our genes, a legacy from times when calories were harder to come by, when "pointless" caloric expenditures in food-scarce environments could prove deadly. I think that's why I love the physical activity of gardening so much. Knowing that my labors will bring fresh, healthy food to the table adds immeasurably to my motivation. I can easily get lost in hours of physical labor among the rows, something that never happens to me on a StairMaster or stationary bike. (Of course, using machines is better than being sedentary and may be the best option for city-bound folk.)

Incorporating a goal—one that at least feels useful—into workouts can make them far more enjoyable. For example, at my home in British Columbia, I make a point of swimming most days to an island in the middle of a lake. The whole swim is not much longer than my standard pool workout, but reaching that island gives me a sense of accomplishment that's often lacking as I log laps at my home in Tucson.

The best thing about integrative exercise is that it's easy to get by doing housework and yard work and, especially, by walking. Walking outdoors with friends is great for emotional well-being. Not only does it give you the mood-boosting effect of physical activity, but it also puts you in touch with nature and provides the added benefit of social interaction.

I know many people who report that regular exercise is the single most effective strategy they have discovered to improve their moods. For example, Kelli, an adoption coach from Redwood City, California, writes:

I have struggled with dysthymia for as long as I can remember—chronic low-level depression with periodic dips to major depressive episodes. Last year after being rear-ended by a very drunk driver, I had to go through my fourth knee surgery and months of recovery. Though the surgery was successful from the standpoint of "fixing" the parts that were injured, I was left with chronic pain. After being frustrated over all that I could not do, I finally shifted to a place where I wanted to focus on what I COULD still do. I found myself drawn to the water, the local YMCA pool to be exact, and started doing lap swimming. I had swum over my life but only as a lark on vacation. Since this was likely now going to be my main cardio activity, I started working to do it properly and for long enough to get health benefits from it. Little did I know this first dip in the pool would lead to a year of now swimming one mile (thirty-seven round-trip laps) four to five nights a week. Not only have I not had a major depressive episode since, but I have dropped twenty-five pounds to boot.

Others sing the praises of running. Depending on your body type, running can either be painful and hard on joints or a fast track to physical and mental transformation. Kim, from Boston, found it to be the perfect way to exit a depressive spiral triggered by divorce:

> People said, take depression medication, etc., but I knew what would work for me. I began to run regularly. I never felt so good. Divorce is life-altering. I used exercise to keep my spirits high and my attitude very positive. I ran almost daily, just to push myself and stay positive about my future. I started at five miles, then worked my way up to run the seven-mile Falmouth Road Race in Falmouth, Massachusetts, in 2009. I then continued and ran the Boston half-marathon two months later and finished with training for the Boston Marathon. All the months of this running was such a release of life's troubles. I took aerobics classes, strength-training classes, and ran a lot! I was the happiest I had ever been.

SLEEP, DREAMING, AND MOODS

People who are contented and serene sleep well. They fall asleep easily, stay asleep, and wake refreshed. Conversely, people who are anxious, stressed, or depressed do not sleep well, and chronic insomnia is strongly associated with mood disorders. These are clear correlations, but what is cause and what is effect is not clear. Most experts agree that sleep and mood are closely related, that healthy sleep can enhance emotional well-being, while insufficient quantity or quality of sleep can adversely affect it.

Studies report that about 90 percent of patients with major depression have difficulty initiating and maintaining sleep. Sometimes the insomnia accompanying depression is so profound that the problem is misdiagnosed as a sleep disorder. And chronic insomnia—on and off for the better part of a year—is a strong clinical predictor of depression (as well as all types of anxiety disorders). Five to 10 percent of the adult population in Western industrialized countries suffer from chronic insomnia, making it another likely contributor to the depression epidemic.

When I am depressed, I do not get good sleep. If I'm stuck in mental rumination, I can't fall asleep, because I can't turn off my thinking mind. And I'm likely to wake early with my thoughts racing. Stress and anxiety interfere with my sleep as well. When I'm in good emotional health, I look forward to a sound night's sleep, fall asleep very quickly, have an active and enjoyable dream life, and wake feeling clearheaded and ready to start my day. Typically, I get eight hours of sleep a night. If I get much less than that or if my sleep is disturbed by nonemotional factors, such as international travel, noise, or too much caffeine too late in the day, I do not feel my best on waking, and if that happens several nights in a row, I am irritable and not able to work or concentrate well.

Surprisingly, there is little experimental research on the connection between sleep and emotions. Most of it involves sleep deprivation: human subjects are observed in laboratories over days or weeks when they are allowed to sleep less than normal amounts (up to 50 percent less, for example). Sleep restriction generally makes healthy people less optimistic and less sociable and more sensitive to bodily pain. One study at the University of Pennsylvania found that subjects limited to four to five hours of sleep per night for one week reported feeling more stressed, angry, sad, and mentally exhausted. Their moods improved dramatically when they resumed normal sleep.

Another study, by investigators at Harvard Medical School and the University of California, Berkeley, used functional MRI to assess changes in brain function with sleep deprivation, in particular the interaction between the medial prefrontal cortex (MPFC) and the amygdala. I've told you that the amygdala is an evolutionarily old brain center that mediates emotional responses to unpleasant stimuli, producing fear and defensive reactions; its activity is heightened in depression. The newer MPFC modulates and inhibits amygdala function to shape more socially appropriate emotional responses; a main finding of the neuroscientific studies of trained meditators is that they have enhanced activity of the MPFC. Sleep-deprived human subjects react more negatively to stimuli, and functional MRI scans of their brains show disconnection of the MPFC-amygdala pathway. This neurological change is one likely mechanism for the effect of sleep on mood. Another might involve cytokines, because sleep deprivation also increases inflammation in the body.

Mood disorders are also strongly linked to abnormal patterns of dreaming and alterations in REM (rapid eye movement) sleep, the phase in which most dreaming occurs. Rosalind Cartwright, PhD, a leading sleep and dream researcher at Chicago's Rush University Medical Center and author of *The Twenty-four Hour Mind: The Role of Sleep and Dreaming in Our Emotional Lives,* has shown that individuals who dream and remember their dreams heal more quickly from depressive moods associated with divorce. Rubin Naiman, PhD, a sleep and dream expert on the clinical faculty of the Arizona Center for Integrative Medicine believes that "REM/dream loss is the most critical overlooked socio-cultural force in the etiology of depression."

Of significance is the fact that most medications used to help people sleep suppress REM sleep and dreaming and also fail to reproduce other aspects of natural sleep. They are some of the most widely used drugs in our society. Many antidepressant drugs suppress dreaming as well. (Those that are stimulants can interfere with sleep in general.)

Research suggests that the emotional content of many dreams is negative. If this is your experience and you find it disturbing, consider Dr. Naiman's view that dreaming is "a kind of psychological yoga," that contributes to emotional wellness. He says that "REM/dreams in the first part of the night appear to process and diffuse residual negative emotion from the waking day; dreams later in the night then integrate this material into one's sense of self." Just knowing that dreams have value can be helpful. Brad, a friend who lives in Phoenix, told me:

> Realizing that dreaming, rather than sleep per se, is vitally important has led me to a perceptual shift that's been very valuable. After hearing a talk by Dr. Naiman about the importance of dreaming, I stopped tormenting myself with thoughts of "I need to sleep," which paradoxically kept me awake with anxiety. Instead, I tell myself, "I need to dream," and surrender easily to the sleeping/dreaming state. I used to fear the negativity of my dreams—it just seemed like useless torment, and staying awake was my subconscious attempt to avoid it. Now that I know that even negative dreams provide a useful release, I embrace them, and I am finally sleeping better. My dreams are getting better, too.

I'm happy to report that my dreams are overwhelmingly pleasant. Often I'm traveling in exotic lands, having great adventures with friends and interesting strangers. My parents, both deceased, are frequently in my dreams, always appearing young, healthy, and in good spirits. Recalling my dreams when I wake can put me in a good mood at the start of a day. I think I owe some of my active and entertaining dream life to melatonin. I take it most nights both for its effect on sleep and dreaming and for its useful influence on immunity. Fortunately, one does not develop tolerance to melatonin as with other sleep aids, and it rarely has negative side effects. (In part 3 of this book, I'll tell you how to use it as part of a program to optimize your emotional well-being.)

The message I want you to take away from these pages is that you must assess your sleep if you want to experience better moods. If you have difficulty sleeping or are not getting enough sleep or sleep of good quality, you need to learn the basics of sleep hygiene, make appropriate changes, and possibly consult a sleep expert. I give specific suggestions on page 207.

EFFECTS OF MOOD-ALTERING DRUGS

Alcohol and Caffeine

The most widely used mood-altering drugs in our society are alcohol and caffeine, the former a "downer," the latter an "upper." (That's depressant and stimulant in medical language.) Both strongly affect mood and behavior and with regular use can lead to dependence and addiction. If you use either and want to attend to your emotional well-being, it is important to look at your relationship with the substance and learn how it might be affecting your moods.

It may seem odd that depressed individuals would be drawn to a depressant drug, but that is the case. Alcohol first affects the inhibitory centers of the brain, causing alertness; confidence; feelings of energy, warmth, and excitement; good mood; and dissipation of anxiety—a welcome, if temporary, respite from stress and sadness. The disinhibition it causes accounts for its perennial popularity as a social lubricant at cocktail and dinner parties and romantic encounters. It is worth deconstructing the term *happy hour* for an alcohol-centered get-together at the end of the day, especially with coworkers in a restaurant or bar that offers drinks at discounted prices during certain hours. Not only does it equate happiness with the effect of a mood-altering drug, but it restricts the experience of it to a particular situation and implies that happiness is not to be had in all the hours of the day without alcohol.

In larger doses, alcohol dulls pain, both physical and emotional, but when it wears off, the pain returns, now accompanied by the physical and mental symptoms of alcohol's toxicity. It is tempting to try to find relief by consuming more. People suffering from depression can easily slide into frequent and excessive drinking to avoid emotional pain, only to become addicted to alcohol and suffer all of the physical, emotional, social, and behavioral consequences of that addiction.

If you use alcohol regularly and are prone to depression or simply want to experience greater emotional resilience and well-being, I would ask you to examine your relationship with it. Ask yourself these questions:

- Do you use alcohol to mask anxiety, sadness, or other negative feelings?
- Do you look forward to the time of day when you drink as the time when you'll feel best?
- Do you depend on alcohol to help you through social situations or periods of increased stress?
- Are you able to experience contentment, comfort, and serenity when you are not using alcohol?
- Do you regularly use any other depressant drugs, such as anti-anxiety or sleeping medications? If so, be aware that their effects and risks are similar to those of alcohol and additive when taken together.

Alcohol can be a benign and useful social/recreational drug that may benefit overall health by reducing stress and the risk of cardiovascular disease. Moderation and awareness are the keys to using it successfully and protecting yourself from harm and the risk of dependence.

Caffeine, especially in the form of coffee, is so much a part of our culture that most users are completely unaware of how powerful a drug it is and how much influence it has on both emotional and physical health. Sensitivity to caffeine varies greatly from person to person. Some people who drink one cup of coffee a day are physically addicted to it, will experience a withdrawal reaction if they cut it out, and have any number of physical and emotional symptoms caused by it (that they probably do not connect to their coffee use). Others can drink many cups a day without any of that.

People like caffeine because it gives them temporary feelings of increased energy, alertness, and focus; many cannot start the day without it. Few understand that the energy provided by coffee, tea, cola, yerba maté, etc., is not some gift from "out there." It is your own energy, stored chemically in your cells, that caffeine prods your body into releasing. When the drug wears off, you are left with a depletion of stored energy and are likely to feel fatigued and mentally dull. As with other stimulants, if you take more caffeine at this point, you can stave off the downside of the drug's effect for a bit, but you run the risk of becoming dependent on it. When people are addicted to coffee or other forms of caffeine, their energy is usually bunched up early in the day and depleted later.

Caffeine makes many people anxious and jittery. Again, in sensitive people, this can occur with small doses. I advise anyone suffering from anxiety, nervousness, and mental restlessness to eliminate all forms of caffeine in order to determine how much it is contributing to those problems or obstructing their efforts to control them. The drug also commonly affects sleep for the worse. I have seen cases of chronic insomnia resolve when patients cut out one morning cup of coffee. Of course, these were very caffeine-sensitive individuals; none of them imagined that an ordinary cup of coffee at breakfast could interfere with falling asleep or staying asleep at night.

Even more interesting to me are the case reports I have collected of people who experienced improvement in mood when they stopped using caffeine. Here, for example, is a letter I received from a friend, Bill, a filmmaker and facilitator from Victoria, British Columbia:

> As far as I can remember, I've experienced some form of depression most of my adult life, although I only became really aware of it through the daily mirroring of a twenty-year marriage. The defining

part of my experience was this "ledge" I would all too easily slip over, sending me into an almost immobilized state.

I never bought into prescription antidepressants. Tales of their side effects kept me away. So, I started with alternatives like St. John's wort, which worked reasonably well but never completely tackled the problem. For the longest time, coffee—three large cups every morning—seemed to help. The caffeine appeared to keep me "up," but what went up also went down: the price was a huge dip in my energy in the afternoon. After a few years passed, I was back to the usual tendencies.

Recently, I slipped into a deeper depression than I had experienced for a long time. In the midst of it, I just happened to see a post on Facebook about alternative mood cures and clicked on the link. The first thing I read was that coffee was more a contributor than cure. I immediately went cold turkey off of it. What followed were three or four mentally foggy days and some headaches. Ibuprofen nipped most of them in the bud. On another recommendation, I started taking daily doses of two supplements, 5-HTP and L-tyrosine, to balance my serotonin levels. Almost immediately, the "ledge" seemed to disappear.

Now, over a month later, while still in the midst of life's trials and inconsistencies, I find myself down at times, but it feels more like a natural state and passes quickly. I have dropped the supplements and satisfy my caffeine yearnings with occasional high-quality black tea. I have more energy, healthier sleep, and a better interface with friends, associates, and daily challenges.

My friend's experience is typical and revealing. Many people consider coffee to be a mild antidepressant, because it can boost mood when used occasionally or when used regularly by those who are less caffeine-sensitive and resistant to its addictive properties. In people dependent on their stimulant effects, coffee and other caffeinated beverages may well be more contributory to depression than counteractive.

The only way to know how caffeine may be affecting your moods is to stop it completely. Note whether you have a withdrawal reaction: fatigue and throbbing headache are the most common symptoms, but digestive upsets and other reactions may occur; these usually appear by thirty-six hours after the last dose of the drug, persist for two to three days, and are instantly relieved if you put caffeine into your system. If you have such a reaction, this is proof that you have been addicted to caffeine and an indication that it has probably affected your energy level, sleep, and moods. See how you feel without it.

Be aware that you may be getting more caffeine than you think, because it is in many products, not only the familiar beverages and chocolate but also decaf (!), energy formulas (drinks, shots, powders, and pills), non-cola sodas, herbal products, diet pills, and over-the-counter cold, headache, and pain remedies. To do the experiment properly, you will need to eliminate all caffeine from your life.

"Recreational" Drugs

Most drugs that people use to alter their moods, perceptions, and thoughts are either depressants or stimulants. Barbiturates (Seconal, Nembutal, "reds"), Quaaludes, and opiates all depress brain function, while cocaine, methamphetamine, and ephedrine stimulate it. Frequent or regular use of any depressant or stimulant drug can lead to dependence and addiction and undermine emotional health and stability. If you are in the habit of using substances of this sort and want to improve your emotional well-being, I advise you to learn about their effects, see how your moods change if you discontinue them, and seek professional help if you have difficulty separating yourself from them.

Cannabis (marijuana) is neither a depressant nor a stimulant but can also have significant cognitive and emotional effects. There is a great deal of individual variation in responses to cannabis. Some people find that it relaxes them, makes them more sociable and less angry, increases sensory pleasure, and helps them concentrate. It works well for some as a natural remedy for pain, muscle spasm, and other medical problems. Others become anxious or paranoid when they use it. It helps some people sleep and keeps others from sleeping. It does not cause the kinds of dependence and addiction associated with stimulants and depressants, but heavy users may consume it every day throughout the day. Although the medical safety of cannabis is great, habitual use can be a factor in suboptimal emotional well-being. If you use it more than occasionally and are going to follow the program in this book, I suggest abstaining from it for a while to find out whether it makes it easier or harder for you to maintain serenity, resilience, contentment, and comfort.

Prescription and Over-the-Counter Medications

Commonly prescribed medical drugs can affect mood, often for the worse. Too frequently, neither the doctor who prescribes them nor the patient who takes them is aware of that potential. For example, antihistamines make many people depressed. (Recall that Thorazine and other major tranquilizers that are used to manage psychotic patients were developed from antihistamines.) Growing up, I had a bad seasonal allergy to ragweed, for which I was given various drugs of this sort. It was a no-win situation for me: either I would be subject to the dismal mood caused by the antihistamines or I would suffer from the allergic sneezing and itching. The drugs made me feel as if a gray curtain had descended over my brain. Although I've lost my allergies as a result of changing my diet and lifestyle and have not needed to take antihistamines in years, I have tried newer versions that are not supposed to get into the brain or cause sedation. I'm sorry to report that they still dampen my mood.

Other big offenders are sleeping and anti-anxiety medications, particularly the benzodiazepines (Valium, Halcion, Klonopin, Xanax, Ambien, Ativan, etc.). These drugs are addictive, interfere with memory, and commonly cause mental clouding and depression. Some experts call them alcohol in a pill. Opiates such as codeine, Demerol, and Oxycontin, which are prescribed as cough suppressants and treatments for chronic pain, are strong depressants. I mentioned the risks of hormones and corticosteroid drugs like prednisone at the beginning of this chapter. With long-term use, steroids cause emotional instability, mania, and, most often, depression. Bronchodilators—used to manage asthma and chronic obstructive pulmonary disease—are strong stimulants that make many people anxious, jittery, and sleepless. Some medications used to control high blood pressure also have negative effects on mood. In fact, so many different kinds of pharmaceutical drugs can influence your emotional life that you should pay attention to any changes you notice when starting on a prescribed medication. I also suggest that you search the Internet for full information on possible psychological effects of any medications you take regularly. Good sites are WebMD.com, drugs.com/sfx, and drugwatch.com.

The same goes for OTC (over-the-counter) products, especially sleeping aids; cough, cold, and allergy remedies; diet pills; and analgesics (pain relievers).

Herbal Remedies

Herbs that affect mood include depressants like kava and valerian and stimulants like ephedra, guaraná, and yerba maté. Occasional use is not a concern, but if you take any of these regularly, pay attention to their effects on your emotions. Other natural products sold online, in health food stores, groceries, and pharmacies may contain psychoactive substances: read labels carefully.

In summary: many commonly used beverages; prescribed, OTC, and recreational drugs; as well as herbal and natural remedies affect mood. Frequent or regular use of them can make it harder to attain optimum emotional well-being and get maximum benefit from the program I have developed.

Exposure to Light

In 1974 I moved from Tucson, Arizona, to Eugene, Oregon, where I thought I wanted to live. I had a community of friends there and loved exploring the majestic forests of the nearby Cascade Mountains. I made the move in June, when the Arizona desert was unbearably hot and summer in western Oregon was delightful. With the coming of fall, the reality of living in a rain forest hit me. Not only was it the wettest place I had ever lived, it was the most sun-deprived. Yes, I found beauty in the pearlescent light that filtered through the low clouds and mist most days, but I began to long for the bright sun and blue skies of southern Arizona. As the days got shorter, my energy dropped, and with it my mood. I don't consider myself particularly weather-sensitive. I welcome cloudy days and storms in the desert because rain is so welcome there, but I came to learn that I cannot go too long without sun.

One friend of mine gets depressed if she experiences more than two sunless days in a row. People like that are not hard to find, and it's been known since ancient times that many people get the blues in winter, particularly in the Nordic countries, where "winter depression" is common. (Interestingly, Iceland is an exception, probably because its inhabitants have unusually high tissue levels of omega-3 fatty acids from a diet rich in oily fish, as well as high dietary intake of vitamin D, also from fish.) In 1970, Herbert Kern, an American research engineer who suffered from winter depression, wondered if lack of light was the cause and if treatment with light might help him. He got the interest of scientists at the National Institute of Mental Health, who came up with a light box designed to approximate bright daylight. Within a few days of treating himself, Kern found that his depression lifted.

In 1984, Norman E. Rosenthal, MD, and colleagues at the National Institute of Mental Health described a form of depression that recurred seasonally, usually in winter, was more common at higher latitudes and in women, and was accompanied by distinctive symptoms such as increased appetite for and intake of carbohydrate foods and weight gain. They called it seasonal affective disorder (SAD) and documented it in a controlled study using light-box therapy. Initially met with skepticism, Rosenthal's ideas are now validated; his 1993 book, *Winter Blues,* is the classic treatise on the subject. The DSM-IV recognizes SAD as a subtype of major depressive episodes. An estimated 6.1 percent of the US population suffers from SAD, and more than twice as many people are prone to a milder form called subsyndromal seasonal affective disorder, or SSAD.

Although many mechanisms have been proposed to explain seasonal slumps in mood—including changes in hormones and neurotransmitters—most experts consider light to be the critical factor. Evolutionary psychologists argue that SAD is an adaptive response akin to hibernation, a way to conserve energy by reducing activity in the most food-scarce seasons in generally food-scarce environments; in women it might have played a role in regulating reproduction.

Whatever its cause, treatment with full-spectrum light—not the same as ordinary indoor light—works to relieve SAD as effectively as antidepressant drugs and faster. It has been so successful that some people have also tried it for nonseasonal depression and other mood disorders. There are not many well-designed studies of light therapy, but analysis of data so far suggests that it can be effective for treating nonseasonal depression, again working as well as medication.

I do not have SAD or SSAD, but I find that daily exposure to bright light contributes to my emotional well-being. I concur with experts who say that to get the best possible sleep, our bedrooms should be completely dark and we should get some exposure to bright light during the day. Natural sunlight is best. I wear UV-protective sunglasses when I'm outside to reduce my risks of cataract formation and macular degeneration. (These do not have to be dark or even tinted. You can get clear protective lenses that block both UV and retina-damaging blue wavelengths.) I also wear a hat and put sunscreen on my face and bald head, but I expose the rest of my body to the sun when I swim. I pay attention to the angle of the sun in the sky and stay out of it when its harmful rays are most intense.*

Light affects our moods, and I urge you to get outdoors frequently. I have never used a light box or other light-therapy device. Several different designs are on the market, some portable, at a wide range of prices. If you live at a high latitude, you might consider adding light-box therapy to the other recommendations I give you, but I must also give you one caution. Many devices include wavelengths of blue light that are hazardous to the eye, increasing the risk of age-related macular degeneration (AMD); that condition is the most common cause of blindness in older people. People who find light-box therapy beneficial may be harming their retinas. (Herbert Kern, the engineer who first tried it, reported in an article in *Science* in 2007 that the treatment became less and less effective for him as his eyesight deteriorated from AMD. "Now I can hardly see," he wrote, "and all hell has broken loose....I have had periods of depression lasting over a year.") Blue light with wavelengths in the 460- to 465-nanometer range is most dangerous and does not appear to be necessary for light therapy to be effective. Newer products claim to deliver light that is free of harmful wavelengths. Shop carefully.

ANTIDEPRESSANT DRUGS: WHEN TO USE THEM

If you suffer from major depression, you may have to take prescribed antidepressant medication. Let me caution you again that the approaches described in this section and in the overall program in this book are not substitutes for antidepressant drugs in the management of severe forms of depression. Used together with medication, they may enable you to

---

* The sun's rays are most harmful between 10 a.m. and 3 p.m. throughout the year; nearer to the summer solstice; closer to the equator; at higher altitudes; and near reflective surfaces like snow and sand.

get by with lower doses of the drugs, shorten the duration of treatment with them, and make it easier to transition off them.

The reason to exercise caution with antidepressant pharmaceuticals is simple: their actions in any one person are impossible to predict. For Nancy, fifty-five, a lawyer, they proved quite valuable:

> Going through a divorce, I tried my typical coping strategies, such as talking with trusted friends, reading self-help books, prayer, listening to music, drinking alcohol, eating chocolate, and regular, vigorous exercise. I could not feel anything but overwhelming sadness. I sought the help of a therapist, who suggested I try antidepressants in addition to talk therapy and occasional tranquilizers. She also taught me self-hypnosis, meditation, talking to "the empty chair," writing letters never to be sent, journaling, and deep breathing. I was on antidepressants for about a year. I was afraid of them at the beginning. I worried that, assuming they worked, I would never be able to stop taking them, that if I stopped, I would get depressed again.
>
> At first, I did not like how I felt on the drugs. Everything was slightly removed, like I was living life through a filter. I was afraid to be on them, and afraid to get off. But once my emotional juices started flowing again, there was no stopping them. I felt everything— even things I had never felt before. I think the antidepressants really helped me. I don't understand the chemistry, but as time passed, it was like they woke me back up. I climbed out of that black pit, and at some point I started feeling joy again. The therapeutic activities in combination with the medication worked for me. After about a year I was weaned off the antidepressants (with a little trepidation). Thankfully, I can report that everything stayed OK. This was twenty-five years ago.

On the other hand, some people find taking antidepressants an almost entirely negative, even nightmarish, experience. Jacqueline, forty-five, a teacher from Westlake Village, California, writes:

I have tried many medications for my depression/mood disorder and have found that I am extremely sensitive to them, and react most severely to antidepressants. After two extremely bad reactions (anxiety, deep depression, suicidal ideation) in two months, I was hospitalized. Soon after, I began to look for alternative therapies. I began to see a doctor (MD) who also specializes in natural remedies. With his help, I have improved greatly. Some examples of the vitamins and supplements I take are vitamin D, B-50, fish oil, L-lutein and SAMe.*

Given this variability in individual response and potential for adverse reactions, I asked Dr. Ulka Agarwal, a California psychiatrist who is studying to be an integrative mental health practitioner, how she uses these drugs to ensure that the benefit will outweigh the risk. This is her reply:

I consider prescribing antidepressants to anyone whose functioning is impaired either socially, occupationally, or academically — are they having trouble getting out of bed and to class or work on time? Can they focus and concentrate? Are they motivated to get through their daily activities? What is self-care like? Are they withdrawing socially or from previously enjoyed hobbies/activities? Does anything bring them joy anymore? Is their sleep disturbed? Are they having suicidal thoughts? If they are impaired in several of these areas or suicidal, I will recommend an antidepressant. In addition to the medication, I recommend weekly therapy, daily exercise, and stress management (yoga, meditation, sports, contact with animals, etc.). I also ask them to eliminate or reduce alcohol and drug use (I work at a university health center, so many of my patients smoke marijuana regularly) and discuss sleep hygiene. I have not yet incorporated nutrition, supplements, or herbal treatments into my practice but hope to soon.

---

* S-adenosyl-L-methionine, pronounced *sammy,* is a naturally occurring molecule.

I usually start with an SSRI, especially if there is some associated anxiety, anger, irritability, or bulimia, but my medication choice depends on the specific symptoms and the side effects of the medication. For someone with decreased appetite and/or poor sleep, I might try mirtazapine (Remeron, a tetracyclic), which induces appetite and is sedating. My first choice for SSRIs is usually Prozac, since it is the least likely in its class to cause weight gain, is not sedating for most people, and is easy to taper off due to its long half-life.

For an isolated or first episode of depression, I recommend treatment for at least six months. If the person has had previous episodes of depression or has done poorly off antidepressants in the past, I recommend nine to twelve months of treatment.

I always taper patients off medications, even Prozac, never stop them suddenly. I usually write out a week-by-week taper schedule.

These are sensible guidelines. If you are taking antidepressants or considering taking them, please keep these points in mind:

- You may not need to be on medication for the long term, particularly if you are working to improve your overall emotional well-being. Ask your physician about when and how to try discontinuing a prescribed drug.
- Long-term use of antidepressant drugs may actually prolong depression, a very concerning problem recently termed "tardive dysphoria" (lingering bad mood). When exposed to drugs that increase serotonin levels at neural junctions in the brain, the body responds by making less serotonin and dropping serotonin receptors, changes that do not quickly reverse when the drugs are discontinued.
- Never stop taking antidepressants without discussing it with your physician, and never stop them abruptly. Taper off them gradually, following a recommended schedule.
- Different types of antidepressants have different actions and different side-effect profiles. Pay attention to both positive and negative

effects of these drugs and report them to your physician. If you do not get significant benefit within eight weeks or you can't tolerate the side effects, it may be worthwhile to consult a clinical psychopharmacologist to select the medication that is best for you.

- Recent research suggests that antidepressant medications may increase the risk of heart attack and stroke in men and breast and ovarian cancer in women. These are tentative findings; pay attention to this line of research if you use the drugs.
- Remember that for mild to moderate depression, many treatment options exist other than prescription antidepressants.

ANTI-ANXIETY DRUGS: NOT RECOMMENDED

I have a low opinion of all the drugs prescribed for anxiety. They interfere with memory and cognition, can worsen mood, and are addictive; withdrawing from them can be very difficult. Furthermore, they do not get at the root of anxiety; they merely suppress it. They may be okay for occasional use to manage acute anxiety, but I strongly advise against taking them frequently or regularly or relying on them to deal with chronic anxiety.

The most powerful and effective anti-anxiety measure I know is the quick and simple breathing technique that I explain in the next chapter (see page 145). I have seen it work for the most extreme forms of panic disorder, when the strongest medications failed. It is perfectly safe, requires no equipment, and costs nothing. And, unlike suppressive drugs, it undoes anxiety at its root.

I address anxiety in patients also by suggesting lifestyle adjustments, particularly with regard to intake of caffeine (and other stimulants), physical activity, stress management, and sleep. For some, I recommend cognitive therapy and meditation practice (discussed in the following chapter) and often suggest trials of valerian and kava (see below) as alternatives to prescribed drugs.

NATURAL REMEDIES FOR DEPRESSION AND ANXIETY

Do an Internet search for natural depression remedies and you'll find a *lot* of stuff for sale: vitamins, minerals, herbs, amino acids, and more, singly and in combination formulas. I'm sorry to tell you that few of these products have been studied systematically and even fewer in well-designed human studies. There is little hard evidence to support the claims made for most of them by manufacturers, practitioners, and patients. I've told you that there is very good evidence for the efficacy of fish oil and vitamin D to boost and maintain emotional wellness, and weaker evidence for a few of the B-vitamins. The natural remedies below are treatments for depression and anxiety rather than preventives, and I do not recommend them for everyone, as I do with fish oil and vitamin D. I think they are worth trying for specific emotional problems as alternatives to pharmaceutical drugs. They can be taken singly or in combination. Some can be used along with antidepressant drugs, others not or with caution. If you get benefit from them, I suggest that you try to taper them off gradually over several months to see if you can maintain improvement in mood without them.

St. John's Wort

This European plant *(Hypericum perforatum)* has a long history of medicinal use, including as an herbal mood booster. It is by far the most studied alternative treatment for depression, and most experimental results with mild to moderate depression have been positive, with St. John's wort performing better than a placebo, often doing as well as prescription antidepressants, and sometimes proving more effective than the drugs. There is no good evidence that it works for severe depression. I would never recommend St. John's wort as a stand-alone treatment to anyone with a diagnosis of major depression.

We still don't know just how this herbal remedy works. Two active compounds have been identified, hypericin and hyperforin, which may affect the serotonin system in the brain. St. John's wort is generally safe but may increase sensitivity to sunlight, may have an additive effect with SSRI antidepressants, and may change the metabolism of other drugs. The last possibility is of special concern to people on birth control pills, immunosuppressants, some cancer and HIV medications, and blood thinners. If you are on any prescribed drugs and want to try a course of St. John's wort for mild to moderate depression, discuss possible interactions with your physician or pharmacist.

Peter, fifty-five, a teacher from Strafford, Missouri, found that after taking St. John's wort for the first time, the effects were rapid and positive:

> It's supposed to take three weeks or so to "kick in" and be fully effective. I took one in the evening and then forgot about it. Next morning I came downstairs and found my depression had disappeared. I forgot all about the herb I had tried and asked my wife what I might be doing different today that was helping me. She looked at me and we both said "St. John's wort!" at the same time!
>
> I thought this must be a placebo effect, but I've taken it off and on several times since, and whenever I get back on the herb, I find almost immediate results in the lifting of depression. Now I stay on it all the time and find the results very good. Instead of one pill three times a day, I take two pills twice a day because this seems easiest for me.
>
> I love that it has no side effects. As a former stockholder of the company that makes Prozac, I am most impressed with the safety of this herb!

However, for most, the onset of benefits comes more slowly. Jean, sixty-eight, a retired registered nurse from Borlange, Sweden, writes:

I am an American woman, married to a Swedish man, and living in Sweden for the past ten years. Five years ago, my forty-one-year-old autistic son died quite suddenly from status epilepticus. His death left me feeling very broken and alone. After a return to the States for his funeral and time to grieve with the rest of the family, I returned to Sweden.

I expected to feel normal grief and sadness for some time, but when it continued, and indeed deepened after about six months, I decided that I needed some help in recovering. I was taking several medications for hypertension at the time, and was reluctant to add yet another pharmaceutical to the mix.

I decided to try St. John's wort, which is a well-accepted therapy for depression here in northern Europe. I took 300 milligrams of the remedy in capsule form, three times a day, and began to feel better within four to six weeks. I continued this therapy for about three years and felt that it was a helpful treatment. It eased the depression, without any noticeable side effects. After that period of time, I discontinued taking it, and felt that there was absolutely no withdrawal.

Look for tablets or capsules standardized to 0.3 percent hypericin that also list content of hyperforin. The usual dose is 300 milligrams three times a day. You may have to wait two months to get the full benefit of this treatment. If it doesn't do much for you after four months, it is probably not worth continuing.

SAMe (S-adenosyl-L-methionine)

A naturally occurring molecule found throughout the body with high concentrations in the adrenal glands, liver, and brain, SAMe has been extensively studied as an antidepressant and treatment for the pain of osteoarthritis. Although the study populations have been small, results have generally been positive, showing SAMe to be more effective than a placebo. In recent research (reported in August 2010 in the *American Journal of Psychiatry*), investigators from Harvard Medical School and

Massachusetts General Hospital gave SAMe or a placebo to seventy-three depressed adults who had not responded to prescribed antidepressant drugs; all continued to take the drugs. After six weeks of treatment, 36 percent of the subjects taking SAMe showed improvement, compared with just 18 percent of the placebo group. Moreover, 26 percent of those in the SAMe group had complete remission of symptoms, compared with just 12 percent in the placebo group.

Carol, sixty-one, of Tucson, Arizona, works for a church. For both her and her husband, the mood lift provided by SAMe was an unexpected side benefit:

> I went through an initial and follow-up visit to your Integrative Medicine Clinic in February 2007, looking for help with osteoarthritis that seemed to be progressing and a number of other challenges. One of the recommendations I received was to take 200 milligrams of SAMe three times a day.... I tried it, and my husband joined me. We began with the recommended dose, and within one day of taking it, we both noticed a huge feeling of well-being. While I can't remember if physically we hurt less, we most definitely saw a difference in our attitudes and felt a feeling of... well, being able to do more.

Janette, forty-eight, from Paradise, California, abused alcohol from her teenage years onward to cope with depression she had felt for "almost my entire life." The prescription antidepressant Trazodone had not worked for her; neither had St. John's wort:

> Through further research, including Dr. Weil's books, I learned about SAMe. I started taking it about five years ago and it has really helped me tremendously. When I first started taking it, I used about 800 milligrams a day and now I use 400. I take it when I feel I need it but can go months without it. I like how it only takes a few days to work. It stabilizes my mood, and I don't feel the severe lows I used to feel. That being said, I also continue to work on myself and grow, and that process

coupled with the SAMe has really helped me. In fact, I no longer drink any alcohol because I don't need it anymore, and my drinking was ultimately very self-destructive. I have been sober for two and a half years.

We don't know how SAMe works; it may affect levels of neurotransmitters or their brain receptors. An advantage of SAMe over prescription antidepressants and St. John's wort is that it works quickly, often lifting mood within days rather than weeks. It is also quite safe, although, because it has been reported to worsen manic symptoms, those with bipolar disorder should avoid it. The only side effect, which is uncommon, is gastrointestinal upset. If you want to try SAMe, look for products that provide the butanedisulfonate form in enteric-coated tablets. The usual dosage is 400 to 1,600 milligrams a day, taken on an empty stomach. Take lower doses (under 800 milligrams) once a day, a half hour before the morning meal; split higher doses, taking the second dose a half hour before lunch. You can use SAMe with prescribed antidepressants (and other medications). It may be especially useful for people who suffer from pain as well as depression.

Rhodiola

Rhodiola rosea, a relative of sedum and jade plant native to high latitudes of the Northern Hemisphere, is the source of arctic root, an herb with a long history of traditional use in Scandinavia, Siberia, Mongolia, and China. It has been valued for antifatigue, antistress, and sexually stimulating effects and has been extensively studied by scientists in Russia and Sweden. Rhodiola root contains rosavins, compounds that appear to enhance activity of neurotransmitters in the brain and may be responsible for the herb's beneficial effects on mood and memory. In a 2007 double-blind, placebo-controlled human study from Sweden, researchers concluded that treatment with a standardized extract of rhodiola showed a "clear and significant antidepressant activity in patients suffering from mild to moderate depression," with no adverse effects.

If you experience mental fog and fatigue along with mild to moderate depression, you might consider a trial of rhodiola. Look for 100 milligram tablets or capsules containing extracts standardized to 3 percent rosavins and 1 percent salidroside. The dosage is one or two tablets or capsules a day, one in the morning or one in the morning and another in early afternoon. This can be increased to 200 milligrams up to three times a day if needed. High doses can cause insomnia, especially if taken late in the day. Interactions with antidepressant drugs, anti-anxiety drugs, and other prescribed medications are not well documented. Pay attention to any undesired effects, such as increased stimulation or anxiety, if you use rhodiola together with pharmaceutical drugs.

Valerian and Kava for Anxiety

Valerian comes from the root of a European plant *(Valeriana officinalis)* used safely for centuries to promote relaxation and sleep. Because the root has a strong odor that many find disagreeable, this herb is best taken in tablet or capsule form rather than as a tea or tincture. Unlike modern drugs used to reduce anxiety and promote sleep, valerian is not habit forming and does not have additive effect with alcohol. The chemistry of this herb is complex, and its mechanisms of action are not known. It is nontoxic.

Use extracts of valerian standardized to 0.8 percent valeric acid. For relief of anxiety, try 250 milligrams (one capsule or tablet) with meals, up to three times a day as needed. This herbal remedy can be used safely with antidepressants.

Kava is another root with a sedative effect, this one from a tropical plant *(Piper methysticum)* related to black pepper and native to islands of the South Pacific, where it has a long history of use as a social and recreational drug. Kava is an excellent anti-anxiety remedy, shown in controlled human trials to be as effective as benzodiazepine drugs. It also is a muscle relaxant.

Because of rare reports of liver toxicity associated with certain types of kava products, no one with a history of liver disease should use this herb. It may have additive effect with alcohol and other depressant drugs; otherwise it is generally safe. You can purchase powdered whole kava root to make into tea or other drinks, but I usually recommend extracts standardized to 30 percent kavalactones. Dosage is 100 to 200 milligrams two or three times a day as needed. Kava works quickly to relieve anxiety, often with one or two doses. Do not use it continually over long periods of time (more than a few months).

Two Ayurvedic Herbs to Know About: Ashwagandha and Holy Basil

Ayurveda is a centuries-old traditional system of medicine that originated in northern India. It promotes health through attention to diet and lifestyle and makes use of a large repertory of medicinal plants, most of them unknown in the Western world until recently. Contemporary research is proving many of them to be safe and effective, some with unique and useful benefits. I consider the two described here to be worth experimenting with.

Ashwagandha, sometimes called Indian ginseng, comes from the root of *Withania somnifera,* a plant in the nightshade family esteemed in India for its tonic and stress-protective effects. The species name *somnifera* means "sleep-bearing," indicating a calming action. Animal research shows ashwagandha to be equivalent to true Panax ginseng in stress protection, without ginseng's stimulating effect. Human studies in India demonstrate ashwagandha's anti-anxiety and mood-elevating properties and confirm its lack of toxicity. If you experience agitation with depression, high stress, and poor sleep, experiment with a six to eight week trial of ashwagandha.

Tieraona Low Dog, MD, one of the world's foremost experts on botanical medicine and a prominent faculty member of the Arizona Center for Integrative Medicine, likes to make a pleasant tonic tea with this herb. She simmers 1 to 2 teaspoons of powdered ashwagandha with 2 cups of milk (dairy or soy) on low heat for fifteen minutes, then adds 2 tablespoons of honey or agave nectar and ⅛ teaspoon of ground cardamom, stirs the mixture well, and turns off the heat. Dr. Low Dog recommends drinking 1 cup of this tea once or twice a day. She also says this:

> Studies in animals show that ashwagandha counters many of the unwanted biological effects of extreme stress, such as prolonged elevation of cortisol and insulin and suppression of the immune system. It also inhibits many of the biochemical mediators that cause inflammation in the body. This makes ashwagandha one of our best plant allies for those who are under chronic stress, not sleeping well, feel tired, and have muscle aches and pains. This describes a considerable number of people that I see in my practice — people who do not meet the criteria for major depressive disorder or generalized anxiety disorder but describe themselves as feeling overwhelmed, exhausted, and tense. They also typically show signs of early arthritis and insulin resistance, and they catch colds frequently. Ashwagandha is perfect for these individuals. It relaxes without sedating, so it can be taken during the day, and is not associated with any known serious side effects. Because quality can vary considerably in herbal products, it is probably best to purchase an extract that has been standardized to contain 2.5 to 5 percent withanolides (key compounds in the root). The dose I recommend is 300 to 500 milligrams taken two to three times per day.

Ashwagandha can be used safely with antidepressants.

Holy basil, or tulsi *(Ocimum sanctum),* is a sacred plant in India, always planted around temples of the Hindu deity Vishnu and often around homes. It is a relative of our culinary basil with a stronger, clovelike aroma and taste. Indians do not use it in cooking but do use it as medicine, mostly in the form of tea. Modern research in both animals and humans demonstrates a lack of toxicity and a variety of benefits. For example, it reduces inflammation and protects the body and brain from the harmful effects of stress. And it has a positive influence on mood (and is safe to use with antidepressants).

My colleague Jim Nicolai, MD, medical director of the Integrative Wellness Program at Miraval Resort and Spa in Tucson, tells me he has had great success with holy basil in his patients:

> I was first introduced to holy basil more than ten years ago, during my fellowship training at the University of Arizona's Center for Integrative Medicine. I read about its antioxidant and anti-inflammatory properties, but what fascinated me more was its use by mystics and meditators in India as a *rasayana*—an herb to foster personal growth and enlightenment.
>
> Holy basil has been shown to lower elevated levels of cortisol, the long-acting stress hormone produced by the adrenal glands. High levels of cortisol can damage the cardiovascular system, retard immunity, create imbalances of other hormones, kill memory cells in the brain, worsen bone loss, increase carbohydrate cravings, raise blood pressure, cholesterol, and glucose, and accelerate the aging process.
>
> Most of my clients have stress-related conditions that I am always trying to help them manage. Holy basil is now at the top of my list of plant-based strategies to target such issues. My personal experience with it is that it lengthens my emotional "fuse"; my reactive fight-or-flight response to stress is much less intense when I take it. I find it gives me greater patience and more opportunity to be mindful. I have been recommending holy basil for the past seven years, and most of my clients swear by it. It is one of the few remedies I'd take with me if I were going to a desert island.
>
> I like holy basil for individuals whose stress levels are causing health problems, and I use it as an alternative to prescription drugs for mild to moderate disorders of mood.

I typically recommend extracts standardized to 2 percent ursolic acid in 400 milligram capsules at a dosage of two capsules one to two times daily with food.

And a Few Words About Turmeric

Turmeric, the yellow spice that colors curry and American yellow mustard, is a potent natural anti-inflammatory agent. Its active constituent, curcumin, has shown promise as an antidepressant in animal models; it also enhances nerve growth in the frontal cortex and hippocampal areas of the brain. Indian researchers suggest doing clinical trials to explore its efficacy as a novel antidepressant. Because turmeric and curcumin offer myriad health benefits, including reduced risk of cancer and Alzheimer's disease, I often recommend them as dietary supplements. They are poorly absorbed from the GI tract, but a recent finding is that absorption is greatly increased by the presence of piperine, a compound in black pepper. Indians—who eat turmeric at almost every meal—get its anti-inflammatory and other benefits because they usually add it to foods along with black pepper. If you want to try turmeric or curcumin supplements as part of this program, look for products that also contain piperine or black pepper extract and follow dosage instructions on labels. You can take turmeric or curcumin indefinitely and combine them with antidepressant drugs or with any of the other herbs and natural remedies I have listed.

OTHER BODY-ORIENTED METHODS — ACUPUNCTURE, TOUCH, HANDS IN DIRT

Acupuncture

A few studies suggest that acupuncture can be a useful treatment for mild to moderate depression. For example, in a controlled trial from

China in 1994, depressed patients treated six times a week with acupuncture for six weeks improved as much as those treated with amitriptylene (Elavil). Study numbers were small, however, and expectations of the benefits of acupuncture among Chinese patients might have produced a significant placebo effect. It is difficult to rule this out because there is no good sham treatment for acupuncture that is equivalent to giving a sugar pill instead of an active drug.

In traditional Chinese medicine (TCM), placement of acupuncture needles is determined by an individual patient's pattern of symptoms and by pulse diagnosis. Different practitioners have different styles. Some studies use electroacupuncture, a nontraditional technique in which pulsating electric current is delivered through the needles. We have no data to suggest a mechanism for how acupuncture might relieve depression, and there is no agreement as to how frequently or for how long it should be done.

I would not recommend acupuncture for severe depression or as a sole therapy for any form of depression. It might be useful as adjunctive treatment, and if you want to try it, look for a practitioner experienced in using it for mood disorders.

The Importance of Touch

Touch can be a powerful contributor to emotional well-being. We know that animal and human infants deprived of physical contact do not develop normally; some actually sicken and die. Now we are learning that touch builds trust between people, allays fear, and helps elicit generosity and compassion. We never outgrow our need to be touched, but, unfortunately, we live in a touch-deprived society. I believe that the lack of touch adds to the social isolation that goes hand in hand with epidemic depression.

Some new, intriguing studies are documenting the biochemical benefits of touch. As reported in a study published in the October 18, 2010, issue of the *Journal of Complementary and Alternative Medicine,* researchers at Cedars-Sinai Medical Center in Los Angeles recruited fifty-three healthy adults; twenty-nine were randomly assigned to a forty-five-minute session of deep-tissue Swedish massage, and the other twenty-four to a session of light massage. All participants had intravenous catheters so that blood samples could be drawn before the massage and for up to an hour afterward.

The researchers found that a single session of massage caused positive biological changes. Those who received deep-tissue massage showed significant drops in levels of cortisol in their blood and saliva as well as drops in arginine vasopressin, a hormone that can boost cortisol. They also generated more white blood cells, evidence of increased health of the immune system. The light massage yielded advantages, too. Volunteers who received it showed bigger decreases in ACTH (adrenocorticotropic hormone, secreted by the pituitary), which stimulates the adrenal glands to release cortisol, and they had greater increases in oxytocin, another pituitary hormone associated with contentment, than did those who received the deep-tissue massage.

For years, oxytocin was thought of only as the hormone that stimulates dilation of the uterine cervix and uterine contractions at the onset of childbirth as well as the production of breast milk soon after. Like all endocrine hormones, however, oxytocin has a broad spectrum of action, including effects on the brain and emotions. It is now commonly referred to as the hormone of love, trust, and pair bonding. Touch promotes the release of oxytocin, which in turn causes the release of dopamine in the brain's reward center. This mechanism may underlie the formation of social bonds and the building of trust between people. The process can start with a simple handshake and go on to activate the same brain systems involved in the emotions of friendship and love.

Paul J. Zak, PhD, a founder of the contemporary field of neuroeconomics, who is both an economist and brain scientist, considers oxytocin to be the "social glue" that helps us maintain closeness with friends as well as an "economic lubricant" that makes people more empathetic and generous. In one experiment in his lab at the Center for

Neuroeconomics Studies at Claremont Graduate University in Claremont, California, half of a group of subjects received a fifteen-minute massage while the other half rested, and then they all played an economic game using real money. In the game, subjects were entrusted with money by strangers in the hope that they would reciprocate. The brains of those who got massage released more oxytocin than the brains of those who rested. And the massaged subjects returned 243 percent more money to the strangers who showed them trust.

I believe that in the realm of touch, variety is key. Just as we need to eat diverse nutrients and engage in a range of physical activities, human beings need a variety of touch experiences on a regular basis. These might include friendly handshakes, hugs, physical contact with companion animals, massage sessions, and passionate sex. As long as both participants engage willingly, there are few experiences that offer human beings a more profound opportunity for improving and maintaining emotional well-being.

Hands (and Nose) in Dirt

I have loved gardening and growing indoor plants since I was a child. For many years now I have raised most of the vegetables I eat in home gardens and also gotten much pleasure from growing flowers and other ornamentals. The mental and spiritual rewards of gardening are many. Here I want you to know about a possible benefit of exposing your hands and nose to dirt, one that might account for some of those rewards through a physical mechanism.

An article with the provocative title "Is Dirt the New Prozac?" in the July 2007 issue of *Discover* magazine reported the results of a study published online in the journal *Neuroscience* in March of that year with a much less catchy title: "Identification of an Immune-Responsive Mesolimbocortical Serotonergic System: Potential Role in Regulation of Emotional Behavior." The lead author, Christopher Lowry, a neuroscientist at the University of Bristol in the UK, became interested in the "hygiene hypothesis," the recently popular idea that living in environments that are too clean accounts for the sharp rise in the incidence of asthma and allergies in developed countries over the past century. Proponents of the hygiene hypothesis argue that excessive cleanliness deprives young people's developing immune systems of routine exposure to harmless microorganisms in the environment, such as soil bacteria. Without this exposure, our immune systems might not learn to ignore such molecules as those in pollen or pet dander. Pursuing this line of reasoning, some researchers have tried treating people with a common and benign soil bacterium called *Mycobacterium vaccae*. Preliminary results indicate that injections of a killed vaccine made from it can alleviate skin allergies. The vaccine has also been found to reduce nausea and pain in some lung cancer patients and, surprisingly, improve their general quality of life and mood.

To determine the mechanism for these effects, Dr. Lowry injected mice with the *M. vaccae* vaccine and also blew killed, pulverized bacteria into their windpipes. He then looked for changes in their brain centers that regulate mood. What he found is that treatment with the bacteria affected cytokine production in the animals and activated serotonin-producing neurons in key brain centers. He concluded that the bacteria "had the same effect as antidepressant drugs." A coauthor of the *Neuroscience* paper, Graham Rock, an immunologist at University College, London, thinks exposure to *M. vaccae* stimulates growth of immune cells that curb the inflammatory reactions underlying allergies. Because depression may be, at least in part, an inflammatory disorder associated with abnormal cytokine activity, exposure to *M. vaccae* might be a novel way to boost mood.

It's a long way from experiments with a few mice to practical recommendations for people who want to be happier, but it can't hurt to kick up some dirt and not be afraid to inhale a little dust when you're digging in the garden. You can also expose yourself to beneficial mycobacteria by eating vegetables fresh from the garden   if you don't scrub off every speck of dirt.

A SUMMARY OF BODY-ORIENTED APPROACHES TO EMOTIONAL WELL-BEING

- Before you start on the program in this book, make sure that you are in good physical health and have no conditions that might be undermining your emotional wellness.
- I've told you that the best evidence we have of the effectiveness of physical interventions to optimize emotional well-being is for supplemental fish oil and exercise. The former is so easy and has so many preventive and therapeutic benefits that I give it high priority. Regular exercise requires motivation and commitment but also is such a key component of a healthy lifestyle that I put it too at the top of the list. Keep in mind that the goal is to get some physical activity every day, that integrative exercise is good for both mind and body, and that getting regular exercise both prevents and relieves mood problems.
- It is easy to take vitamin D and B-vitamins as supplements, harder to change your eating habits. The most important dietary advice I can give you is to stop eating refined, processed, and manufactured foods. Read over the principles of my Anti-Inflammatory Diet in Appendix A and start to incorporate them into your life. Informed food choices can help you reduce overall risks of disease, maintain good health as you age, and help you feel better, both physically and emotionally.
- If you are prone to depression or anxiety or just want to be happier more of the time, I urge you to look at all mood-altering drugs you may use, from caffeine and alcohol to medications and all the other classes of substances discussed in this chapter. They may be affecting your emotional life more than you realize. Experiment with the natural remedies I've listed.
- Pay attention to your sleep and dreams and learn what you need to do to improve them. Sleep in complete darkness and try to be out in bright light during the day. And find ways to satisfy the need for physical touch to promote contentment and comfort.

6

Optimizing Emotional Well-Being by Retraining and Caring for the Mind

Most of us think of the mind as the home and source of our emotions, even though we commonly experience them in the body as well. We get choked up with emotion in the throat and go with gut feelings; fear gnaws at the pit of the stomach; we sense love and heartache in the chest. The fact is that our dynamic emotions pervade the unitary body/mind, mediated by an elaborate network of nerves, neurotransmitters, and hormones. If you want to increase your emotional resilience or move your emotional set point toward more positive moods or simply want to be more open to the possibility of spontaneous happiness, you can use methods directed at the body, as described in the previous chapter, or methods directed at the mind, or, better, both.

Who has not tried to cheer up a depressed friend or family member by offering reassurance, love, or just a sympathetic ear? Some of us need only to talk out our troubles to stop ruminating on them and feel better; innumerable varieties of talk therapy are available to serve this need. Many of the mental health professionals who offer it identify depressive rumination as a root cause of unhappiness. This is the tendency to brood over a few characteristic negative thought patterns and lose control over the thinking process, so that depressive ideas keep intruding and crowding out others. As I told you at the end of chapter 2, evolutionary psychologists propose that so many of us tend to engage in depressive rumination because evolution has selected it as a useful trait. They argue that depression makes sense as a problem-solving mode that spurs us to withdraw and deeply contemplate some thorny issue or situation. Ideally, it is self-limited. Either the brooding leads to discovery of a solution, or, if there is no solution, it should abate when at some deep level we sense that the situation can't be helped and decide to move on.

Unfortunately, the process often goes awry and plunges people into lasting misery. When you are stuck in depressive rumination, you can't stop chewing on your problems, which may be as vague and insoluble as "I am a loser." There is no end point. No one seems to know why this happens; the usual mix of genetic, lifestyle, and social factors is probably responsible. The practical challenge is how to get unstuck.

I've told you that when I'm depressed, I can't fall asleep, because I can't turn my thinking mind off. This is also the case when I'm worried, and I'd like to share with you some insights I have about worrying as one variety of ruminative thought that does us no good. Both *rumination* and *worry* have root meanings associated with the mouth, the former with chewing the cud, the latter with obsessive biting, as a dog worries a bone. *Worry* comes from an Old English verb meaning "to strangle or kill" in the way a predator seizes its prey by the throat, shakes it back and forth relentlessly, and does not let go. That is an arresting image, one that gives the word a deep meaning.

Anyone who has raised a puppy knows the chewing phase that can be so trying. My first Rhodesian ridgeback entered it one day, as if some circuit were suddenly activated in her developing brain. She would go into chewing frenzies focused on any convenient object, including me. Once, when I was trying to deflect her attention from my hand to a stick, we locked eyes, and I saw in hers a look that conveyed total helplessness in the face of an overpowering neurological drive. It was as if she were saying, "I don't want to be doing this anymore. It's wearing me out, but I can't stop. Help!" I could empathize with her distress at being unable to turn off her chewing and biting, to stop worrying every object she mouthed, because I could relate her helplessness to my own experience of inability to stop ruminating over thoughts that make me anxious or sad.

Mark Twain advised to "drag your thoughts away from your troubles...by the ears, by the heels, or any other way you can manage it," but managing thoughts might be one of the most difficult challenges for human beings. Our minds produce thoughts in continuous streams, as if from an engine whose controls are not accessible to us. Of course, some of these streams are very useful. They help us navigate the world and can make us feel more comfortable with ourselves and more content with our lives. I am certain, however, that a great deal of the fear, anxiety, and despair that people suffer arises from negative thoughts.

Until recently, Western psychology tried to alleviate this kind of emotional pain by making people aware of how they came to develop such thoughts—for instance, by remembering incidents of abuse or failure in early life that might have started the patterns. Sigmund Freud identified the unconscious mind as the repository of repressed painful memories that spawn neurotic patterns of thought and behavior. Psychoanalysis, the classic method he developed to integrate the mind, is extremely time- and cost-inefficient; the most succinct and trenchant criticism of it I have heard is this: "When you've got a poisoned arrow in you, you don't need to know how it got there; you want to know how to get it out." Freudian psychoanalysis is today very much out of fashion, but most of the styles of therapy that have evolved from it have also focused on bringing to light the *why* of negative thinking without giving people practical tools to change it.

Almost a century after Freud, radically new forms of psychotherapy have become popular in the Western world. Practitioners of positive psychology and cognitive psychology teach people how to modify the process of thinking and replace negative thoughts with positive ones. I am most enthusiastic about these new methods.

POSITIVE PSYCHOLOGY: INTERVENTIONS TO TRY

Though it is rooted in the humanistic psychology of the 1950s, an independent branch of the field known as positive psychology is quite recent. Its chief proponent is Martin Seligman, PhD, of the University of Pennsylvania, who convened the first positive psychology summit in 1999.

Seligman launched the movement because he was dismayed that traditional psychology aimed only to make "dysfunctional people functional." Accessing the higher, happier realms of human emotion—contentment, engagement, gratitude, joy—was generally deemed trivial, impossible, or otherwise too far outside the realm of therapy even to attempt. Seligman felt this attitude was foolish: why exclude the better half of human experience from the world of psychology? Why be content to make dysfunctional people functional if you could make people happy?

Seligman observed that those who tend to get depressed following setbacks in life differ from others in how they explain such events to themselves. They take them as confirmation of lack of self-worth, instead of seeing them merely as temporary reversals of fortune. This difference in explanatory styles turns out to be the key difference between optimists and pessimists. Furthermore, Seligman's research showed that people can *learn* to be more optimistic by consciously reworking their styles of interpreting what happens to them. His discovery echoes philosophical teachings of the ancient world. For example, the Greek philosopher Epictetus (55–135 CE), who taught mostly in Rome and based his work on that of the earlier Stoics, advocated transformation of the self to attain a state of happiness or flourishing *(eudaimonia)* by making proper use of impressions. What he meant by *making proper use of impressions* was reinterpreting sensory experience so as not to have automatic negative emotional reactions. He taught: "Remember that foul words or blows in themselves are no outrage, but your judgment that they are so. So when anyone makes you angry, know that it is your own thought that has angered you. Wherefore make it your endeavor not to let your impressions carry you away."

This teaching is a cornerstone of positive psychology. We cannot always control what happens to us, but we can learn to control our interpretation of what happens to us and in so doing learn to be more optimistic and feel better about ourselves. I find this to be a process requiring attention and practice. Like most authors I know, I consider articles and books that I write to be extensions of myself and tend to take criticism of them personally. During the years when I was prone to dysthymia, I made my living as a writer, often doing commissioned pieces for magazines. To have an article rejected by an editor was devastating. I took it as a rejection of *me* and would let it plunge me into a long period of despair in which I would ruminate over my failings not only as a writer but as a person. Epictetus would have said that I let my impressions carry me away and, as a consequence, prevented myself from experiencing happiness and being my best. With practice, I have learned to reinterpret rejections and criticism of my creative work as annoyances that have no impact on my self-esteem. I also try to consider them dispassionately to see what I can learn from them. This change—still in process—has spared me a great deal of emotional grief.

Rather than focusing on ways to identify and eliminate negative thoughts, Seligman designed therapeutic exercises—termed *interventions*—to spotlight and enhance a patient's positive emotions. The interventions of positive psychology seek to boost three basic types of happiness:

- pleasure, which includes sensory enjoyments such as delicious food or passionate sex
- flow, the sensation of being wholly absorbed in a task that is neither too easy nor too demanding

- meaning, the overall fulfillment that stems from using your highest strengths in service to something larger than yourself

From its modest recent beginnings, the field of positive psychology has grown rapidly, with its own professional journal, popular and academic books, and an annual international conference. Together with like-minded colleagues, Seligman has tested many interventions to help people enjoy greater pleasure, flow, and meaning in their lives and has found three to be particularly effective. The Gratitude Visit, in which the participants write down and recite essays of gratitude to persons who have been kind to them, causes an immediate spike in happiness, but the effect tends to dissipate after a month. Two others have more lasting impact. The Three Good Things intervention has the participant write down each day for a week three things that are going well and the reasons why; it can lift happiness for a full six months. The Using Signature Strengths intervention, in which the participant takes a test to identify his or her personal strengths, such as creativity or forgiveness, and uses a "top strength" in a new, different way daily for a week, also yields a six-month mood improvement.

Many who have experienced these and other positive psychology interventions are enthusiastic about the results. Petrina, thirty-seven, an occupational therapist from Hamilton, Ontario, Canada, writes:

> I have lived with depression since I was quite young, and over the years I have learned that my ability to reframe my thoughts has a tremendous influence on my mental health. I first encountered positive psychology through the book *Authentic Happiness* by Martin Seligman, and I found it to be quite helpful. In all the reading I had done on depression, this was the first that took a truly strengths-based approach to happiness. And while I am the first to acknowledge that medication, cognitive-behavior therapy, and other disease-focused therapies are incredibly important for treating conditions like mine, I am so thankful to Dr. Seligman for offering an

alternative perspective. I feel that it gave me the opportunity to accept more of the whole story of who I am, and it suggested a means for developing skills, a perspective, and a lifestyle that focused on keeping me well rather than simply addressing what was going wrong with me.

And Brenda, forty-nine, a therapist from Smyrna, Tennessee, has this to say:

I am a master's level graduate in counseling and have a lifelong history of depressive symptoms, treatment, and personal as well as professional research on depression. Positive psychology has been the most effective tool I've found for managing my periods of depression. Arriving at this point was through epiphany-like experiences that thankfully I was open to enough to receive, even through the fog of symptoms. There is so much to it, my experiences with aspects of positive psychology, but the one key helpful part is staying in the present moment and therefore fully experiencing what is happening now, which also leads to creating good feelings by using gratitude and hopefulness. There is joy to be had if we just are open to it.

As you can tell, I'm a great fan of positive psychology. I agree wholeheartedly with Seligman's assertion that much modern unhappiness springs from the "society of the maximal self," which encourages an obsessive focus on the individual rather than on the group. Numerous studies show that the happiest people are those who devote their lives to caring for others rather than focusing on themselves. That's why many of Seligman's interventions — such as talking with homeless people, doing volunteer work, or spending three hours a week writing fan letters to heroic people — aim to foster selflessness in daily life by creating opportunities to develop empathy and compassion and put the interests of others ahead of your own.

There is profound wisdom embodied in this movement. I urge you to explore it further. While some therapists employ its insights in their work, it is not a formal branch of clinical psychology. The best way to approach it is to read Seligman's book *Authentic Happiness: Using the New Positive Psychology to Realize Your Potential for Lasting Fulfillment,* and try the interventions listed there. You can also find resources at www.ppc.sas.upenn.edu, including exercises that may help you move your emotional set point. Some colleges are teaching positive psychology classes to students, and adult education programs offer courses as well.

One of the best things about positive psychology is that you can choose from its "menu" of interventions to find ones that fit your lifestyle, inclinations, and schedule; some can be done in as little as a week.

COGNITIVE PSYCHOLOGY AND COGNITIVE BEHAVIORAL THERAPY

As a freshman at Harvard College in 1960, I wanted to study what most interested me: consciousness. But shortly after I chose psychology as my major, I realized I had made a mistake. At that time, academic psychology was under the spell of behaviorism and its leading proponent, Harvard's own B. F. Skinner, who became my advisor. Skinner was a highly entertaining and persuasive lecturer, as well as a creative experimentalist; his laboratory work with rats and pigeons gave us the terms *positive reinforcement* and *negative reinforcement.* The goal of behaviorist psychology was to describe, predict, and, ultimately, control behavior (both animal and human) as a function of environmental influences, such as rewards and punishments, without reference to internal mental states that were considered beyond the reach of scientific investigation. In other words, consciousness was excluded from behaviorist psychology and from the psychology department at Harvard, which I found exceedingly frustrating—so much so that I switched my major to botany.

Soon after, although I was unaware of it at the time, the new field of cognitive psychology began to supersede behaviorism. *Cognition* comes from a Latin verb "to know" and refers to the totality of our mental abilities: perceiving, learning, thinking, remembering, reasoning, and understanding. Scientific study of these functions was facilitated by the rise of computers and development of the fields of computer science and artificial intelligence. Although the human mind and brain differ significantly from computers, computers gave psychologists a model for approaching the internal mental states of human cognition. By drawing analogies from the operations of code within computers, cognitive scientists were able to propose ways that our minds work. Ironically, it was experiments with machines rather than with rats and pigeons that led psychologists to embrace consciousness and start to analyze its contents. The new movement caught on quickly and has had great influence. If I were an undergraduate today, I would be much less frustrated: Consciousness Studies is now a legitimate major in many colleges.

Unlike positive psychology, cognitive psychology produced a robust clinical arm. American psychiatrist Aaron T. Beck (1921–), who developed a cognitive theory of depression in the 1960s, is regarded as the father of cognitive therapy. Beck attributed depression to faulty processing of information in individuals who had negative views ("schemas") of the world. There may be a genetic predisposition to this, but Beck believed such negative perspectives often result from rejections, losses, and other traumas in early life. However the schemas develop, they warp thinking in ways that continually reinforce negative bias. For example, depressed persons are quick to overgeneralize and to engage in selective perception and all-or-nothing thinking. They habitually interpret their experience through a distorted lens, letting their impressions carry them away to unhappy realms. (In his original treatment manual, Beck wrote, "The philosophical origins of cognitive therapy can be traced back to the Stoic philosophers." His work inspired that of Martin Seligman.) By making people aware of their cognitive habits and teaching them to substitute alternative ways of thinking and interpreting perceptions, cognitive therapy can relieve depression and restore emotional wellness.

Beck's cognitive therapy (CT) is now one of a number of therapeutic methods within the larger framework of cognitive-behavioral therapy (CBT). A National Association of Cognitive-Behavioral Therapists (www.nacbt.org), formed in 1995, is a large and active organization with more than ten thousand members that certifies practitioners and provides referrals. Membership includes psychiatrists, clinical psychologists, and licensed social workers and counselors who have completed CBT training. Whatever their particular styles, CBT practitioners work from the assumptions that our thoughts cause our feelings and behavior and that we can change the way we think in order to feel better and act better. The rapid growth of CBT is easy to explain. Not only does it work, but it is much more time- and cost-effective than more traditional forms of psychotherapy.

A great many clinical trials show CBT to be effective. In a 2011 publication, the British Royal College of Psychiatrists concluded that CBT:

- is one of the most effective treatments for conditions where anxiety or depression is the main problem
- is the most effective psychological treatment for moderate and severe depression
- is as effective as antidepressants for many types of depression

Patients typically require five to twenty sessions of thirty to sixty minutes, spaced a week or two apart. They first learn the model of CBT and begin to master the skills involved. Depressive symptoms often improve in this initial stage, and many patients are no longer depressed after only eight to twelve sessions. A full course of treatment is fourteen to sixteen sessions, with occasional booster sessions during the following year to maintain improvement. CBT can be done individually or in groups, and people can also get started with self-help books and online programs.

To guide patients toward discovery of the kinds of thinking that make them feel bad about themselves and the world, CBT practitioners use a variety of strategies and methods, including Socratic questioning, role playing, visualization (see page 143), and behavioral experiments. Once patients recognize their negative thoughts, they may be asked to decide whether there is evidence to support them or whether alternative thoughts might better reflect reality. They receive assignments for homework between sessions. Ideally, as cognitive therapy proceeds, the patient will be able to spot distorted thinking when it arises and get in the habit of "reframing" the situation. Although formal therapy hours are few, CBT is not a quick fix. It can make you aware of the faulty thinking responsible for emotional pain and give you the tools to correct it. Then you have to practice the skills you have learned.

A recent innovation is mindfulness-based cognitive therapy, which combines mindfulness training — that is, the practice of bringing all of our awareness to the here and now — with CBT. In a study reported in the December 2010 issue of the *Archives of General Psychiatry,* researchers from the Centre for Addiction and Mental Health in Toronto showed this combined therapy to be as effective as antidepressant drugs in preventing relapses of depression. They studied 160 patients, ages eighteen to sixty-five, who had been treated for major depressive disorder and had two past episodes of depression. All of the patients were given antidepressants until they were symptom free. Then some remained on medication, some received a placebo, and the rest were assigned to mindfulness-based cognitive therapy. Those in the therapy group attended eight weekly group meetings and did daily homework, which included mindfulness practice. The emotional health of all patients was assessed at regular intervals. After eighteen months, the relapse rate in the mindfulness group was about 30 percent, the same as it was for the patients who continued to take antidepressants. In the placebo group the relapse rate was much higher — 70 percent.

I frequently refer patients to CBT and recommend it to you because of the results I have seen. Here is a report from Renée, forty-eight, a social worker in Wichita, Kansas:

> I have done cognitive behavioral therapy and highly recommend it. I used to be a card-carrying pessimist, but thanks to CBT, I have learned to transform my negative thinking. While I still get depressed, I remain optimistic. I know that sounds like a contradiction in terms, but it's really not. I consider the depression to be a physical illness. It runs in my family. But how I choose to react to it is my choice, and I choose to be positive. I usually feel quite depressed physically, but my thought life is very active, positive, and uplifting. I am always learning about my illness and trying to feel better. Learning cognitive reframing and some stress management skills has helped me so much.

Pam, forty-five, a freelance television producer in Los Angeles, has this to say:

> I began suffering from depression at age fifteen—the root cause was maternal neglect and criticism. I suffer from atypical symptoms (overeating, oversleeping, rejection sensitivity). I've been told that I probably suffer from double depression—dysthymia with major depressive episodes on top of it. My depression was severe. I went on disability from work three separate times and felt as though I wanted to die every day of my life. Medication has kept me alive but did not erase the damage that I needed to repair. I began therapy several years ago and saw several PhD therapists who largely utilized psychodynamic techniques. That mode of therapy was virtually useless in treating my depression, as I already had a good understanding of the underlying conflicts that contributed to it. It wasn't until I began seeing an MFT [marriage and family therapist] who utilized cognitive behavioral techniques that I began to heal and experienced relief from my depressive symptoms. Some of the helpful aspects were

treating negative thinking, catastrophizing, automatic thoughts, and negative self-talk. For the first time in thirty years of suffering from chronic, unremitting, and debilitating depression, I finally am in remission and have been for one year. Had I known to seek a therapist who utilized CBT early on, I might have been able to avoid years of suffering.

CBT may not be for everyone, and it may not be right for you. It seems most suited to those who are comfortable with introspection and are willing to use scientific method to understand the workings of the mind. And of course, you have to accept the basic tenet of cognitive psychology, that thoughts produce our moods and behaviors. I find that theory convincing and useful. If you suffer from depression or anxiety or just want to have more control over your shifting emotions, I urge you to try CBT. It represents a great advance in Western psychology's ability to improve emotional well-being.

MEANWHILE, EASTERN PSYCHOLOGY has tackled the challenge of managing thoughts in quite different ways. Advanced practitioners of yoga and Buddhist meditation claim to be able to actually stop thought and free their minds to experience the highest states of consciousness.* Most of us will never be able to do that, but what we can do is break the habit of paying constant attention to our thoughts. Both yogic and Buddhist philosophers see this as a true addiction, one that causes much suffering. Objects of addictive behavior appear to have great power over us. Drugs, food, gambling, and sex can seem so fascinating and attractive that some of us cannot free ourselves from their apparent hold and cannot form healthy relationships with them. Either we indulge in them to excess, often harming ourselves as a result, or we try to abstain from them (not an option, of course, in the case of food).

---

* This state is known as *samadhi* in yoga, *satori* in Zen Buddhism.

Early in my professional career, I studied drugs and addiction and became known as an expert in addiction medicine. I came to see addiction as a widespread and fundamental human problem, deeply rooted in the mind and very difficult to treat. Because some forms of addictive behavior—to shopping, for example, or to accumulating wealth or to falling in love—are socially acceptable, we do not see them for what they are and so do not see how many people struggle with addiction.

Options for the treatment of addiction are few. One can try to modify addictive behavior in ways that reduce its potential for harm, such as going from shooting heroin to oral methadone maintenance, or switching from compulsive overeating to compulsive exercising, or one can try to solve addiction at its root. The former method is practical, the latter very hard. Solving addiction at its root is hard because it demands restructuring of the mind at its core, where we experience the distinction between conscious awareness and the objects of awareness, between the perceiving self and what is perceived.

When people cannot stop reaching for the next snack chip or the next cigarette, it is as if chips and cigarettes control attention and behavior. In reality, the mind gives its power and control to the objects of addictive behavior. Freedom from addiction comes with awareness of that process and the ability to experience the object as object, without projecting onto it any undue significance. This is the essence of the Buddhist teaching that suffering comes from attachment, and to reduce our suffering, we must work to reduce attachment. Furthermore, Eastern psychology insists that thoughts are best experienced as objects of awareness, just like trees or birds in the world around us. We suffer emotional pain because we cannot stop attending to our thoughts, cannot stop seeing them as part of us and habitually giving them great significance. Yoga masters and Buddhist teachers recommend a variety of methods to break our attachment to thoughts. Some are practices intended to shift the focus of attention to something else—to the breath, for example, or to images in the mind's eye, or to sounds. Others aim to develop the power of attention and increase voluntary control of it or to promote awareness of the important distinction between the self and thoughts.

I should mention that talk of stopping thoughts or detaching from them makes some people in our culture uneasy, even terrified. Intellectuals and academics who base their careers and livelihoods on clever and creative thinking may equate these goals of Eastern psychology with losing one's mind. If you have such concerns, you might do better with Western therapies that train you to modify thought without denying the validity or importance of thinking. Personally, I find both approaches effective. Just as I have found value in integrating Western and Eastern medical philosophies in my work as a physician, I have found it useful to combine Western and Eastern psychological approaches to tackle the challenge of managing thoughts that produce anxiety and despair and prevent us from enjoying spontaneous happiness.

Let me review the Eastern methods that have helped me and that I recommend most often to others.

MANTRAM

Mantram (or *mantra*)* refers to the practice of silently repeating (in the "mind's ear") certain syllables or phrases. It is a way to distract the mind from thoughts, putting attention on sounds or words believed to have spiritual significance and positive effects. Most often associated with Hinduism, Buddhism, and other Eastern religions, it is also a Western religious practice, as exemplified by the Roman Catholic Rosary and the Jesus Prayer of the Eastern Orthodox Church.** The most common Hindu mantram is the syllable *aum* (or *om*), representing the essence of the universe; the most common Buddhist formula is

---

* The Sanskrit word is variously translated as "instrument of thought" or "tool for the mind."
** "Lord Jesus Christ, Son of God, have mercy on me, a sinner."

om mani padme hum, a Sanskrit phrase referring to the "jewel in the lotus [of the heart]," a symbol of enlightenment. Suitable phrases are available from nearly all spiritual traditions, from Native American to Jewish.

Some contemporary psychologists, however, recommend mantram as a purely secular method of diverting attention from troublesome thoughts in order to reduce anxiety, anger, and stress. One spiritual teacher and author of books on meditation, the late Eknath Easwaran (1910–1999), likened repetition of a mantram to the bamboo shaft given to elephants in festival processions in India to keep them from grabbing anything they can as they go through the narrow passages of street markets:

> The elephant steps right along with his stick held upright in a steady trunk, not tempted to feast on mangoes or melons because he has something to hold on to. The human mind is rather like the trunk of an elephant. It never rests…it goes here, there, ceaselessly moving through sensations, images, thoughts, hopes, regrets, impulses…. But what should we give it to hold on to? For this purpose I recommend the systematic repetition of the mantram, which can steady the mind at any time and in any place.

Using Easwaran's *The Mantram Handbook,* several researchers have documented the efficacy of this method to improve emotional well-being. One study, published in the *Journal of Continuing Education in Nursing* in 2006, measured outcomes of a five-week program of mantram practice in a population of health care workers (nurses and social workers, primarily female), who were experiencing high stress. Participants were asked to choose a mantram from recommended sayings from the major spiritual traditions and were given wrist-worn counters to tally the daily frequency of repetition. They were asked to practice mantram repetition first during nonstressful times, such as before falling asleep, "to promote an association between the word and a physiological state of calm." They were also taught concepts of one-pointed attention ("focused concentration on the mantram in the mind or on a selected task or activity of one's choice, without multitasking") and of slowing down ("living intentionally without hurry"). Then they were instructed to use the mantram whenever they felt stressed. The investigators found that the program reduced stress and improved the emotional and spiritual well-being of the participants. They concluded that "mantram repetition is an innovative stress-reduction strategy that is portable, convenient, easy to implement, and inexpensive."

Other researchers have come to similar conclusions after testing mantram repetition in male veterans and HIV-positive individuals. Participants learned to use the practice to interrupt unwanted thoughts and elicit a relaxation response. Most reported that they found it helpful in a variety of stressful situations. This accords with my experience. After reading about mantram in my early thirties, I began repeating *om mani padme hum* to myself when I was falling asleep, driving long distances, or just sitting quietly. After a time, I found I could use it to break cycles of worrying that made me anxious or kept me awake. It has also helped me get through dental procedures and remain calm in the midst of turmoil. I do not repeat the words on any fixed schedule or keep count of the number of times I do it, but I've done it so often that I can now slip into it almost without conscious effort. Because mantram repetition is, indeed, portable, convenient, easy to implement, and inexpensive, I recommend it to you as a method worth trying to take your attention away from thoughts that make you anxious or sad.

VISUALIZATION

Another alternative to thought as an object of attention is mental imagery. Visual imagination is powerful. It is mostly what we focus on when we daydream, and it can totally fascinate us when we engage in sexual fantasy. A significant portion of the brain, the visual cortex, is responsible for processing data coming from the retinas and optic nerves. When it is not occupied with that task, it is free to generate pictures of its own and act as a conduit between the conscious and unconscious mind, giving access to parts of the nervous system that regulate circulation, digestion, and other body functions normally considered involuntary. Meditation on visual images is a religious practice in Hinduism and Buddhism, where geometric designs of spiritual significance are used.* After studying these designs, practitioners learn to recall them in the mind's eye. Apart from its religious purpose, this sort of meditation is said to calm the mind and body. (C. J. Jung incorporated the use of mandala into his psychoanalytic work with patients; one Jungian analyst, Gerald Schueler, writes that "chaos in our lives can be transformed into order by the psychic process of drawing a mandala, a universal psychic symbol for order.")

Visual images that we pay frequent attention to can determine the set point of our emotions just as habitual patterns of thought can, possibly more so because they influence physiology so strongly, evoking visceral responses associated with feelings. To get a sense of their power, close your eyes and picture a lemon wedge, freshly cut and glistening with juice. Concentrate on making the image as clear and detailed as you can. Then visualize bringing the lemon to your lips, sucking on it, and biting into it. As you do this, chances are you will experience sensations in your mouth and salivation, just as if you had sucked on an actual slice of lemon. Or consider how rapidly visual fantasy can lead to sexual arousal. Practitioners of visualization therapy and interactive guided imagery teach patients to modify health conditions by taking advantage of this mind/body phenomenon, often with good results. Over the years, I've referred many patients to such therapists and have seen improvement in problems ranging from atopic dermatitis (eczema) and autoimmunity to cancer and recovery from surgery.

---

* These designs are called *yantra* in Hinduism and yoga, *mandala* in Buddhism.

For the purpose of optimizing emotional well-being, I recommend experimenting with visualization in two ways. The first is to practice shifting attention from negative thoughts to mental images that evoke positive feelings. The second is to select an image that you associate with your most positive moods and focus on it frequently. For example, think of an actual place where you experienced contentment, comfort, and serenity. Re-create that scene in your mind's eye, and each time you do, concentrate on sharpening the detail, making the colors brighter, even imagining sounds, physical sensations, and scents that might have been part of the experience. Keep that image as a place you can go to in your mind whenever you feel stressed, anxious, or sad. One place I visit in this way is a secluded pool in a small canyon in the Rincon Mountains east of Tucson, Arizona, where I have had many happy hours lying on polished rocks, dipping into the clear water, being soothed by the sound of running water and awed by the scenery of the Sonoran desert. Even if I am in a New York City subway or a traffic jam in Beijing, I can take myself there in a heartbeat just by closing my eyes. Then I can reconnect with the contentment I experienced there.

BREATH WORK

Putting your attention on your breath is another way to take it off your thoughts. The breath is such a logical and safe object of attention that it is the most commonly used focus of meditation. The more you can train yourself to shift attention away from emotionally upsetting thoughts (or images), the better off you will be, and the breath is a very safe place to shift it — rather like putting your mind's engine in neutral.

Breath links body and mind, consciousness and unconsciousness. Working with the breath is one of the main components of yoga for three reasons. First, it gives access to the involuntary nervous system and makes it possible to influence cardiovascular, digestive, and other functions ordinarily beyond conscious control. Second, it is a way to calm the restless mind, facilitating one-pointed attention and meditation. Third, it promotes spiritual development and well-being, a subject I will return to in the following chapter.

For many years, I have taught medical students and doctors the importance of breath and the practical utility of breath control to improve physical and emotional well-being. I have also taught most of my patients and many thousands of others the simple rules of breath work:

1. Put your attention on the breath whenever possible.
2. Whenever you can, try to make your breathing deeper, slower, quieter, and more regular.
3. Let your belly expand outward when you inhale.
4. To deepen breathing, practice exhaling more air at the end of each breath.

The correlation between breathing and emotions is a dramatic example of mind/body unity. When people are anxious, angry, or upset, their breathing is *always* rapid, shallow, noisy, and irregular. Slow, deep, quiet, regular breathing simply cannot coexist with emotional turmoil, and it is much easier to learn to regulate the breath than to will negative moods to end. The most effective anti-anxiety measure I know is a quick and simple breathing technique that I call the 4-7-8 breath. Here it is:

1. Place the tip of the tongue against the ridge behind and above the front teeth. Keep it there through the whole exercise.
2. Exhale completely through the mouth (and puckered lips), making a *whoosh* sound.
3. Close the mouth and inhale deeply and quietly through the nose to a (silent) count of 4.

4. Hold the breath for a count of 7.
5. Exhale through the mouth to a count of 8, making the same sound.
6. Repeat steps 3, 4, and 5 for a total of four breaths.

This can be done in any position; if seated, keep the back straight. Do this exercise at least twice a day and, in addition, whenever you feel stressed, anxious, or off center. Do not do more than four breaths at one time for the first month of practice but do the exercise as often as you wish. After a month, if you are comfortable with it, increase to eight breaths each time and gradually slow your counts down. The minimum practice is then eight breaths twice a day, every day.

With practice, this will become a powerful means of inducing a state of deep relaxation that gets better over time. It will enable you to stop anxiety in its tracks and will convince you that you have the ability to control your reactions to potentially upsetting events and situations without relying on drugs or other external aids. You need only spend a few minutes a day on this practice, but you must do it at least twice a day without fail. By imposing this rhythm on your breathing with your voluntary nerves and muscles, you will begin to influence your involuntary nervous system toward more balanced functioning, with great benefits to overall health. Making the 4-7-8 breath part of your daily routine will increase your experience of serenity and comfort and give you greater emotional resilience. I have found it enormously helpful in stabilizing and improving my moods, and I cannot recommend it highly enough.

Developing Attention and Concentration

Apart from their value as practical methods of detaching from troublesome thoughts, mantram, visualization, and breath work provide opportunities to learn about attention. Attention is a tool of the mind. Think of it as a roving searchlight that brings to conscious awareness whatever it illuminates. We can direct our attention to objects both internal and external, and sometimes objects seize our attention. Unless we have had appropriate training, however, we often let our attention wander from one thing to another without maintaining its focus on anything for more than a few moments. Like light, attention becomes powerful when it is concentrated. Just as a magnifying lens can concentrate the energy of sunlight to ignite a fire, so can a focused mind concentrate attention to produce extraordinary effects. It is such one-pointed attention that is the secret of mastery of any craft, skill, or performance and of doing anything well, whether driving a car, cooking, or speaking in public. We all know the experience of being so absorbed in a task or activity that we lose track of time and become oblivious to almost everything except what we are doing, but few of us have learned how to develop that sort of attention in a systematic way.

"A Wandering Mind Is an Unhappy Mind" is the title of a report in the November 12, 2010, issue of the journal *Science* about an experiment conducted by two Harvard psychologists, Matthew A. Killingsworth and Daniel T. Gilbert. They developed an iPhone app that contacted 2,250 volunteers aged eighteen to eighty-eight at random intervals to ask how happy they were, what they were doing, and whether they were thinking about their current activity or something else. On average, the subjects' minds were wandering 47 percent of the time and never less than 30 percent of the time (except when they were making love). Other findings were that people were happiest when making love, exercising, or engaging in conversation, and least happy when they were resting, working, or using a home computer—namely, situations that favor mind wandering. Describing the study, one of the researchers said, "Mind-wandering is an excellent predictor of people's happiness. In fact, how often our minds leave the present and where they tend to go is a better predictor of our happiness than the activities in which we are engaged." Furthermore, time-lag analyses of the subjects' responses suggested that their mind-wandering was the cause, not a result, of their unhappiness.

Concentration literally means "gathering (something) to a center." What we gather up when we practice one-pointed attention is conscious awareness. Instead of letting it diffuse aimlessly and drift into the unreality of past memories and future fantasies, we collect it and bring it together in the reality of the present. This is the essence of mindfulness. As I explained in chapter 4, mindfulness training is now widely offered; today, many health care professionals, including mental health practitioners, are using it as part of integrative treatment. There is no downside to learning to be more mindful. Not only can it help you deal with medical and emotional problems, but it can also make you more efficient and skillful in anything you undertake, improve your relationships, and allow you to experience life most fully—all the result of getting better at concentrating and focusing your attention. I encourage the physicians and allied health professionals who train at the Arizona Center for Integrative Medicine to cultivate mindfulness, and I often refer patients to mindfulness-based stress reduction (MBSR) programs. You can find a great deal of information on this form of meditation, derived from Buddhist practice, in self-help books and online, including web-based instruction.

MEDITATION

Mantram, visualization, and breath work are all forms of meditation. Meditation is nothing other than directed concentration—holding the focus of attention on some object. Although many Westerners associate it with Eastern religions, there are Jewish, Christian, and Islamic forms of meditation, as well as purely secular ones intended to reduce stress and evoke the relaxation response. In Buddhist psychology, as distinct from religious Buddhism, meditation is emphasized as a powerful way to restructure the mind, which I find very relevant to the subject of this book. More than just a technique of detaching from unwanted thoughts, meditation can allow you to witness the productions of your mind, including thoughts, from a disinterested, nonattached, nonjudgmental perspective.

The modern spiritual teacher Eckhart Tolle puts it succinctly:

If you can recognize, even occasionally, the thoughts that go through your mind as simply thoughts, if you can witness your own mental-emotional reactive patterns as they happen, then that dimension is already emerging in you as the awareness in which thoughts and emotions happen — the timeless inner space in which the content of your life unfolds.

The stream of thinking has enormous momentum that can easily drag you along with it. Every thought pretends that it matters so much. It wants to draw your attention in completely.

Here is a new spiritual practice for you: don't take your thoughts too seriously.

Meditation is certainly not a quick fix for anything. It is a long-term solution to the core problem of confusing awareness with the objects of awareness (including thoughts) and suffering as a result of attachment. In chapter 4, I told you that after forty years of practice, I still find it hard to meditate and maintain my focus of awareness on the here and now, noting thoughts and sensations as they arise without judging them or reacting to them. I also told you that making meditation a daily habit, shortly after waking in the morning, has been one of the ways I've kept my tendency to dysthymia in check. I wrote about the value of meditation in my first book, *The Natural Mind*, back in 1972, and I have continued to write and teach about it ever since.

Because practicing meditation can contribute greatly to an integrative program for optimum emotional well-being, I recommend that you give it a try. If you find the associations of meditation with religion in general and Eastern religions in particular an obstacle, look for books, audio programs, online instruction, or classes that teach purely secular forms. Simply sitting still and practicing keeping your attention on your breath is a tried-and-true method that anyone can do. Do it even for ten minutes a day, every day, and you will begin the process of restructuring your mind in a way that will bring you greater contentment, serenity, comfort, and emotional resilience.

I HAVE GIVEN you a menu of options for managing thoughts that make you depressed or anxious and get in the way of spontaneous happiness, options from both Western and Eastern psychology. But caring for the mind means more than dealing with your thoughts. In the following pages, I will discuss other mental factors that influence your moods and tell you what you can do to control them.

SOUND AND NOISE

Sound has a direct and powerful influence on the nervous system and on our emotions. We become alert and often anxious when we hear sirens, people arguing, screeching tires, and wailing babies. A lullaby can soothe us and induce sleep. Chanting can focus attention and facilitate meditation. Most people are unaware of the effects of sound on the body and mind, even in the midst of the noise pollution so characteristic of cities and workplaces. I cannot exclude from this chapter information about protecting yourself from disturbing sounds and exposing yourself to sounds that make you feel good.

The most obvious correlations are with anxiety and insomnia. If you suffer from either, I urge you to pay attention to the sounds in your environment and find out how they might be affecting you. Two simple experiments are to turn off televisions and radios if you are not actively listening to them, and to notice how different kinds of music make you feel.

Music powerfully affects the brain and mind. It can make us calm or excited, can stir us to action or paralyze us with fear. If you are unaware of this power of music, you are likely to be careless about exposing yourself to kinds of music that worsen moods. It is all too easy to listen unconsciously to sounds that drive the nervous system away from calmness and centeredness.

In his compelling recent book, *In Pursuit of Silence: Listening for Meaning in a World of Noise,* essayist George Prochnik tells a story of going on patrol with a Washington, DC, police officer named John Spencer:

> All of a sudden, at about three in the morning, Officer Spencer turned to me and said, "You know, I'll tell you something. The majority of domestic disputes we get called into these days are actually noise complaints." What did he mean? I asked. "You go into these houses where the couple, or the roommate, or the whole family is fighting and you've got the television blaring so you can't think, and a radio on top of that, and somebody who got home from work who wants to relax or sleep, and it's just obvious what they're actually fighting about. They're fighting about the noise. They don't know it, but that's the problem. They've just got everything on at once. And so the first thing I'll say to them is, 'You know what, don't even tell me what you think you're fighting about! First, turn down the music. Switch off the game station. Turn down the television.' Then I just let them sit there for a minute, and I say to them, 'Now, that feels different, doesn't it? Maybe the real reason you were fighting is how *loud* it was inside your apartment. Do you still have anything to tell me? Do you?' Well, you would be amazed how often that's the end of it."

If you have ever stayed in Las Vegas—I have attended more than one conference on health there—you know the experience of walking through hotel casinos and being unable to avoid the incessant sounds of slot machines. They take me far away from serenity and comfort, as do many other electronic beeps, pings, and buzzes, not to mention car alarms, leaf blowers, and jackhammers. If you cannot escape disturbing sounds, the new technology of noise cancellation gives you a way to protect yourself from them. Noise-canceling headphones detect environmental noise with built-in microphones and generate signals that neutralize it; they are readily available and affordable. Another possibility, especially useful in the bedroom, is to mask annoying sounds with white noise, which might sound like rushing air or running water. Portable white-noise generators are also readily available and affordable, and there are larger systems that can cover offices and whole houses. Some allow you to select from a range of sounds, from ocean waves to rain.

Apart from neutralizing or masking unwanted sounds, you can, of course, choose to listen to those that have positive effects on your moods. Unlike most electronic sounds, sounds of nature, such as wind blowing through trees and water running over rocks, are complex and may "nourish" the brain in some way. We evolved with the sounds of nature, and the relative lack of them in our artificial environments of today may be yet another cause of emotional malaise. There are many ways to bring healing sound into your living space. I have a set of very large bass wind chimes that make me happy whenever I hear them. The deepest tone has a remarkably long sustain that reminds me of the chanting of Tibetan monks. Whenever I notice it, I tend to close my eyes, focus my attention on my breathing, and let the sound flow through my body. I feel it as well as hear it. It always returns me to my calm center and often brings a smile to my face.

Finally, I recommend cultivating silence as an antidote to the emotionally unsettling effects of sound and noise. I will give you suggestions about that in the next chapter.

MENTAL NUTRITION

Exercising control over the sounds you let in is one aspect of what I call mental nutrition. We know a great deal about nutrition and health in regard to dietary choices and their influence on well-being and risks of disease. Most people, however, do not consider that what we allow into our minds is as important as what we feed our bodies and significantly influences our emotional well-being. It makes sense to be as careful about mental nutrition as about your diet.

If you habitually and unconsciously listen to sad music, read sad stories, and watch sad movies, chances are you will be sadder than if you choose happier input. If you habitually tune in to news programs that make you angry and distraught, chances are you will spend less time in the zone of serenity and contentment. The challenge is to exercise conscious control over what you pay attention to. The world is both wonderful and terrible, beautiful and ugly. At any moment one can *choose* to focus on the positive or negative aspects of reality. Without denying the negative, it is possible to practice focusing more on the positive, especially if you want to shift your emotional set point in that direction.

I advise you to take particular care with your choices of media. A great deal of the content is designed to induce excitement and tension. Often it exacerbates anxiety and the sense of being overwhelmed and out of control. I made "news fasting" a major component of my 8-Week Program for Optimum Health: start by excluding news in any form for one day a week and work up to total abstinence for an entire week. I've had much fun talking about the benefits of this strategy on national television news shows. (Not a few newscasters have told me privately that they wish they could do it.) A great many people who have done it report decreased anxiety and worry and increased happiness as a result of limiting their intake of news. With news actively foisted on us, it takes effort to keep it out of our consciousness. I very much resent being forced to listen to it in hotel elevators and at airport gates. And just as I started to write this, I received an unsolicited e-mail from an acquaintance recommending a website that allows you to click your mouse on any city on a world map and see the day's headlines in the local newspaper.* "Double click and the page gets larger," gushes the sender. "You can read the entire paper from some cities if you click on the right place. You can spend forever here." Just what we all need.**

I will tell you some of the ways I control input to my mind. I pay attention to the effects on my mood of what I read, watch, and listen to for entertainment. I don't watch television except when I'm on the road, and when I'm in a hotel room and flip around the ever-increasing number of channels, I am dismayed by how few acceptable options there are. I have no interest in shows about police and criminals. I do not care for mindless sitcoms and game shows, and I do not tune in to the news. I will watch documentaries: biography, nature, history, and science programs; and I look at the food channels from time to time. I do not read newspapers or newsmagazines but may scan Internet headlines or listen sporadically to National Public Radio. I never worry about being uninformed. If something important happens, someone always lets me know about it. When I sense that I am vulnerable to a slump in mood, I take extra care to nourish my mind well.

I am not an arbiter of taste, and it is not my place to tell you what to read, listen to, or watch. I just want you to be aware that the decisions you make about all of this affect your moods and emotions for better and worse. I urge you to make them mindfully.

---

* www.newseum.org/todaysfrontpages/flash/
** Recently, a number of "good news" sites have appeared on the web, such as www .happynews.com and www.goodnewsnetwork.org. The best one is www.odewire.com. I don't recommend getting all your news from such sites, but it may be worth adding one of them to your Favorites list as an antidote to the negativity that dominates most news outlets.

LIMITING INFORMATION OVERLOAD

News fasting is one way to control the amount and kind of information that comes into your life. Unfortunately for all of us, it hardly has an impact on a much bigger problem of quite recent origin that has serious implications for mental health and emotional wellness. We are told that we are living in the Information Age, that the revolution in collecting and disseminating information made possible by computers, the Internet, e-mail, mobile phones, and digital media is the defining characteristic of our times and the main force now shaping the evolution of human society. I agree. The problem is that a great deal of that information is irrelevant or suspect, and the sheer amount of it is drowning us. In addition, the media that deliver it to us are changing brain function, not necessarily for the better. In chapter 2 I wrote that of all the ways the modern environment and our genes are mismatched, I would cite the revolution in communication and information delivery as the one contributing most to epidemic depression.

Many scholarly articles are in print about information overload and its physical, psychological, and social consequences. Francis Heylighen, a cyberneticist* at the Free University of Brussels, in a 2002 article titled "Complexity and Information Overload in Society: Why Increasing Efficiency Leads to Decreasing Control," writes:

> We get much more information than we desire, as we are inundated by an ever growing amount of email messages, internal reports, faxes, phone calls, newspapers, magazine articles, webpages, TV broadcasts, and radio programs.... The retrieval, production and distribution of information [are] infinitely easier than in earlier periods, practically eliminating the cost of publication. This has reduced the natural selection processes, which would otherwise have kept all but

---

* One who studies communication and automatic control systems.

the most important information from being transmitted.... The result is an explosion in irrelevant, unclear, and simply erroneous data fragments. This overabundance of low quality information has been called *data smog*.... The same applies to the ever growing amount of information that reaches us via the mass media.... The problem is that people have clear limits in the amount of information they can process.

When the amount of information coming at them exceeds those limits, people suffer. They are likely to ignore or forget information they need, be overconfident on the basis of flawed or incomplete information, and be less in control of their lives as a result. In the long term, information overload increases stress, with all of its predictable consequences for physical and emotional health.

I can easily see how my life and the lives of my friends and family have changed with the coming of the Information Age. When I was growing up, both my parents worked, and worked hard, but when their workday ended, it ended, and we could be at home as a family to prepare and eat dinner together, and after cleaning up, read or watch a favorite show on television. Usually I had homework to do for school, and my mother might sew or finish hats for the millinery shop she and my father owned, but our evenings were largely relaxed. With the advent of fax machines, portable phones, computers, and, most of all, e-mail, I found that my workdays never ended; work-related communication and information began to invade all of my waking hours. Then, as the Internet developed and I became more proficient at using it, I no longer needed to go to libraries or consult reference books. Today I can get almost any kind of data I need or want within minutes, sometimes seconds, on my home computer: historical facts, medical references, song lyrics, recipes—just about anything. I can communicate almost instantly with people around the world and do television interviews without leaving my desk. Much of this is great—I can't imagine going back to encyclopedias and snail mail. Unfortunately, I also notice changes that I don't like at all.

For one thing, I experience time passing more quickly. It seems as if the Christmas holidays come around faster and faster, for instance. I know that most people find time speeding up as they age,* but I was quite surprised a few years ago when my daughter, then twelve, told me she and her friends had the same experience. I remember time passing ever so slowly when I was her age; summer vacations seemed very long, and Christmas did not come around before I was ready for it. I think it is information overload that has altered our subjective sense of time by giving us more data to process moment by moment, hour by hour, day by day. There is more happening per unit of time, more to attend to. As convenient and useful as I find the new technologies of communication and information, I also blame them for making me feel as if I never have enough time to catch up. Often I am overwhelmed by all the e-mails and calls and messages I have to return and feel frantic by midafternoon. I find that I don't have—or *take*—time to read as much as I did in the past and that I must force myself to stop thinking about communications and data processing when I get into bed at night if I am to get restorative sleep.

Clearly, information overload is inimical to focused attention. As I wrote earlier in this chapter, focused attention is the essence of mindfulness and the key to mastery of any activity, as well as a mental skill worth developing in order to be happier. So much information coming at us on so many channels forces us to try to attend to more than one thing at a time—to multitask. A great deal of psychological research suggests that performance suffers when people try to do even very simple tasks at the same time. With more complicated ones—such as driving while talking on a mobile phone—the risks are obvious. The reality is that the human brain cannot attend to two or more tasks simultaneously; at best it can rapidly switch back and forth from one thing to another. It is possible that people can become proficient at this

---

* This is perhaps because each passing year is a smaller and smaller fraction of one's lifetime.

kind of switching and that kids raised on video games and multimedia develop mental skills that older folks (like me) don't. Children of the Information Age may even have better brain function for specific tasks, such as the hand-eye coordination required to win at video gaming. Nonetheless, I observe a collective decrease in attention span in our society, and I see it as another detrimental effect of information overload. For example, when I watch television dramas or contemporary movies, I am struck by the shorter duration of scenes relative to those of the past. And I cannot help feeling that the rising incidence of ADHD (attention deficit hyperactivity disorder) in young people is a manifestation of the same problem.

The new technologies may affect brain activity in other ways, with as yet unknown long-range consequences. How I write has changed as I've adapted to word-processing on a computer instead of composing on a typewriter. A lot of the work of word crafting and revision that I used to do in my head (to avoid having to correct or redo typed pages) I now do on the computer screen. I can't imagine going back to the old, cumbersome way of typing out articles and whole books, but I wonder if I have lost some worthwhile mental ability with the change. I resist using GPS navigation systems in cars, because I like relying on my intuition and sense of direction to get where I'm going and don't want to lose those. A colleague who teaches physics to undergraduates at a large university in a neighboring state tells me he has had to "dumb down" his courses in recent years. He thinks computers and calculators have eroded students' intellectual skills; none of them know how to use a slide rule to solve problems, and some cannot add columns of figures.

I mentioned above that inability to process excessive information can make people feel less in control of their lives. That feeling and an associated sense of helplessness are strongly correlated with emotional disorders, with both depression and anxiety. If you pay the most attention to the aspects of your environment and the world that are dreadful, and you feel powerless to change them, you are not likely to enjoy emotional serenity, contentment, and comfort, especially if you are also feeling overwhelmed and swept along by an accelerating rush of time.

Finally, I fear the Information Age might just as well be termed the Age of Social Isolation. We are spending more and more time interacting with other people virtually or not interacting with them at all as we surf the web and indulge in the many forms of escapist fantasy available through multimedia. Social isolation undermines emotional well-being and predisposes us to depression. We must be proactive to avoid it.

I have learned that the hard way. Shortly after I got my first home computer, a friend introduced me to a challenging game with elements of mystery, quest, and treasure hunt in a world of fantasy. I got hooked quickly and found myself staying up until the wee hours three nights in a row, glued to the screen. The following morning I deleted the software and resolved never to do anything like that again. Years later, however, I had to work hard to break the habit of surfing the web for hours, one engaging site leading to another and another, adding up to a similar waste of time. Finding my peace with e-mail has been even more of a challenge, as it has become my preferred way of communicating and keeping in touch with friends and associates. I now do e-mail almost exclusively on my desktop computer, almost never on my cell phone or notepad. The computer stays in my office, and when I leave my office for the day, usually in the afternoon, I leave it and e-mail behind until morning. I recommend that you make similar rules for yourself, lest e-mail take over your life.

I've had an easier time with cell phones for the simple reason that when they came into my life, I lived in an area with no reception (at the base of a mountain range southeast of Tucson). Although I've recently moved from there, my habit of using my cell phone only when I'm away from home and then sparingly is well developed. My daughter taught me to text a few years ago, but I have no problem saving that for exceptional situations. And I am not tempted by the many apps I could install on my smartphone, which many people find so fascinating and use in ways that remind me of my obsessive web surfing of the past. I have consciously worked to change my relationship with telephones in general. As a result of my training in hospitals, for a long time I found it hard not to pay attention to a ringing phone; I felt compelled to answer, even when I was no longer caring for patients. For years, I would run to the phone whenever it rang—from another room or even from outside, more often than not getting to it just as the caller hung up, and feeling frustrated and angry as a result. When answering machines appeared, I thought they would help, but I grew to dread coming home to a long series of recorded messages. These days I no longer let ringing phones command my attention or draw me away from what I'm doing. I'm comfortable with letting many calls go to voice mail. And I like getting those messages as e-mail attachments. I'd say it's taken me thirty years to get to a good place with telephones.

Research helps explain why we find it so difficult to ignore the digital devices that are ever more prominent in our lives, why it takes so much effort to resist checking e-mail before you go to bed, for example, or disregard the beep telling you a new text message has arrived on your cell phone. B. F. Skinner's experiments with rats and pigeons are very relevant here. When caged animals get the reinforcement of a food pellet in response to pressing a bar or button, how hard they will work for the reward is a function of how it is presented: after a fixed or variable interval of time or after a fixed or variable number of presses. Variable ratio schedules of reinforcement—where the food pellet comes after a certain number of presses but that number varies unpredictably from one reward to the next—control behavior most powerfully. Animals will work themselves to exhaustion when bar pressing is reinforced in this way. That's exactly how slot machines pay off, and humans will work relentlessly to get money from them. I'm afraid the compulsion to check e-mail frequently is comparable. Once in a while you get a reward—maybe news of a business success or a love note or a video that makes you laugh out loud—but rewarding e-mails come in on variable ratio schedules in response to your behavior, which is why it's so hard to stop checking to see if one has landed in your inbox.

Furthermore, the sounds that our digital devices make may stimulate dopamine release in the brain. Recall that dopamine is central to the brain's reward system and our experience of pleasure. As annoying as I find the electronic sounds in casinos, people who love gambling (or are addicted to it) find them pleasurably stimulating. It appears that many people now depend on the dopamine-mediated stimulation provided by personal digital assistants, portable phones, video games, and other devices; without it, they are bored.

I've made Limiting Information Overload a major component of the program I will present in the last section of this book and will suggest other strategies for you to try. There is no one right way to do it, but in order to protect your emotional well-being from the harmful effects of data smog and the new media, I think you must decide how connected you want to be and how much of the time and stick to reasonable limits.

GUARDING AGAINST SOCIAL ISOLATION

I've told you that when I was engulfed by dysthymia, I shunned social contact. I rationalized this behavior by telling myself I was in no shape to be out and about, that I didn't want others to see me so off center and didn't want to expose them to my gloom. In retrospect I see social isolation as both a central symptom of my depressions and a major contributing factor to them. When I closed myself to social contact, I slipped into a default state of depressive rumination: going inward, focusing on my thoughts, and chewing on the same negative ones over and over.

Social interaction supports emotional wellness. People got much more of it when they lived in tribes and real communities; there is much less of it in our modern world. At the beginning of the twentieth century, families were typically larger and more stable, divorce was less common, and relatively few people lived alone. In 1900, only 5 percent of US households were single-person households; by 1995, 10 percent of Americans lived alone, and now that number has increased to 11 percent, or roughly 31 million. Not surprisingly, this trend is linked to an increase in the prevalence of loneliness.

A 2006 study in the *American Sociological Review* found that Americans on average had only two close friends to confide in, down from an average of three in 1985. The percentage of people reporting having not even one such confidant rose from 10 percent to almost 25 percent. One estimate is that 20 percent of people in the United States — about 60 million — feel lonely. Loneliness is common in large cities. Despite being surrounded by millions of others, many city dwellers experience absence of identifiable community. Of course, those in small towns and villages can feel lonely, too, but the sheer number of people with whom one comes into contact every day in a big city seems to work against meaningful interaction and increase the sense of being cut off and alone.

Social isolation and loneliness are strongly correlated with depression. In his classic work, *Suicide,* Émile Durkheim (1858–1917), the father of modern sociology, wrote, "Man cannot live without attachment to some object which transcends and survives him.... [If] we have no other object than ourselves, we cannot avoid the thought that all our efforts will finally end in nothingness, since we ourselves disappear." Of course, existential loneliness is an inescapable part of the human condition, but you have a lot more time to dwell on it if you live in isolation, focused on yourself. Durkheim attributed depression to social isolation and argued that it is one of the common causes of suicide. Recent research on the psychological effects of solitary confinement of prisoners suggests, to put it bluntly, that people lose their minds when they are completely deprived of contact; growing awareness of this truth may one day end the practice of putting prisoners "in the hole" as cruel and unusual punishment.

Researchers have documented an association between Internet use and social isolation as well as depression among adolescents. (It is not clear whether high Internet usage weakens social ties or whether young people with poor social ties gravitate toward Internet activity; I suspect that it works both ways.) Increasingly, lonely people of all ages are flocking to Internet sites to find help or reduce their emotional pain. Put "I am lonely" into a search engine, and you will find many sites that offer virtual interaction with other lonely souls. Maybe this shared electronic space provides some comfort, but I doubt that it offers the emotional protection of the real thing.

For much of my adult life I lived in relatively remote places, often on the borders of wilderness. I enjoyed the rewards of living close to nature, away from noise, traffic, and pollution, but that was at the expense of enjoying much company. Few people wanted to drive so far over rough roads to visit me, and it took a lot of effort to get myself to go into town to spend time with others. I thought I liked it that way, because I'm often on the road teaching, speaking to large audiences, and appearing on television and radio, and when I get back from such trips, I want to hide out. But I've come to realize that my preference for living away from people is not good for me. Writing is a lonely occupation to begin with, and being physically isolated has only made it easier for me to ruminate on thoughts that make me unhappy, no matter how beautiful the scenery. Finally, in my late sixties, I have admitted to myself that I need more quality time with people. I can no longer ignore the fact that my moods are greatly influenced for the worse by social isolation and greatly lifted by social interaction.

In 2010, I put my rural property up for sale and moved into a comfortable house in Tucson, the first time I've lived in a town in almost fifty years. Pulling up roots and moving were difficult, but within a few weeks I began feeling at home in my new place and very pleased that I no longer had such a long drive if I wanted to meet people for a meal or an outing. It is also much easier to invite friends over.

Many aspects of contemporary life promote social isolation. We live in nuclear families, not tribes. We learn to be suspicious of strangers, to look out for ourselves. We have grown accustomed to the impersonal nature of many of our interactions. We are seduced by virtual reality, multimedia, and forms of communicating that merely simulate real contact. If you want to be in optimum emotional health, realize that social isolation stands between you and it. Reach out to others. Join groups—to drum, meditate, sing, sew, read, whatever. Find communities—to garden, do service work, travel, whatever. We humans are social animals. Spontaneous happiness is incompatible with social isolation. Period.

A SUMMARY OF MIND-ORIENTED APPROACHES TO EMOTIONAL WELL-BEING

- Understanding that depressive rumination is a hallmark of depression and that thoughts are the major source of sadness, anxiety, and other negative emotions should motivate you to manage them.
- Read up on positive psychology and select a few interventions that have helped people become more optimistic and happier. Give them a try.
- Familiarize yourself with the theory and methods of cognitive psychology and consider working with a CBT practitioner. CBT is the most time- and cost-effective form of psychotherapy for depression and anxiety.
- If what I wrote about mantram repetition as a tool to interrupt negative thinking interests you, select an appropriate word or phrase and experiment with it to see if it helps.
- Experiment with mental imagery as an alternative focus for your attention. Work with a particular image of a place you associate with positive emotions and focus on that whenever you feel sad, anxious, stressed, or in the grip of negative thinking.
- Whenever you remember to do so, make your breathing deeper, slower, quieter, and more regular. Practice putting your attention on your breath when you find you are stuck on troubling thoughts. Also practice the 4-7-8 breathing technique and use it to control anxiety.

- Develop your powers of attention and concentration. Try to bring more of your awareness to the present moment. Mindfulness training is an excellent way to do this.
- Consider some form of daily meditation practice.
- Identify sounds in your environment that affect you for the worse. Find ways to neutralize or mask them. Expose yourself to sounds of nature and listen to music that makes you happy.
- Exercise greater conscious control over what you let into your mind, especially from the media. Try taking breaks from the news.
- Set limits on the amount of time you spend on the Internet, with e-mail, on the phone, in front of the television, etc. Information overload will get you if you do not take steps to protect yourself.
- Make social interaction a priority. It is a powerful safeguard of emotional well-being.

7

Secular Spirituality and Emotional Well-Being

Most integrative mental health practitioners believe that spiritual life and emotions are linked. Some even argue that depression is primarily a spiritual disorder, one that affects the mind and is associated with secondary changes in the brain and body. As a founder and proponent of integrative medicine, I have long taught that human beings are mental/emotional beings and spiritual entities as well as physical bodies, and that medicine must address *all* aspects of patients to be most effective.

Often, however, I find it awkward for two reasons to discuss spirituality. First, many people confuse spirituality with religion. Although the two may overlap, religion usually demands dogmatic adherence to beliefs that are ultimately not provable, and differences in those beliefs are common causes of suspicion and conflict in our world. Second, spiritual reality concerns the nonphysical aspect of our being. Western science and medicine adhere to the philosophy of materialism, which dictates that only what can be directly perceived, touched, and measured is real; to materialists, the term *nonphysical reality* is an oxymoron.

Let me clarify what I mean by *spirituality* in relation to emotional well-being. I do not mean belief in God or deities, nor do I mean taking anything on faith at the expense of rationality. I do not mean any sort of religious ritual or practice or reliance on "holy" books or people. I do mean acknowledging and attending to the nonphysical, essential self as part of comprehensive self-care. Physicians who train at the Arizona Center for Integrative Medicine learn to include a "spiritual inventory" as part of a complete medical history. It includes such questions as: "What are your main sources of strength?" "If you had a life-threatening illness, where would you turn for support?" "What gives your life meaning and purpose?"

Forget religious uses of the word *spirit*. Ignore the confusion of spirits with ghosts. Think instead about what people mean when they talk about the spirit of something or getting into the spirit of an activity. Why is *dispirited* a synonym for "depressed"? How about the phrase *That's the spirit!* as a commendation for right action?

When I wrote about breath work in the previous chapter, I promised to tell you more about it in this one. From ancient times and in many cultures, Eastern and Western, people have identified breath with spirit; in many languages—curiously not English—the same word means both "breath" and "spirit."* Breath is the *essence* of life— our most vital, core function. When breathing ceases, life ceases. Of course, breath exists in the physical body, and air moving in and out of the lungs is a physical reality. But breath is also insubstantial, a mysterious rhythm that straddles conscious and unconscious awareness, links body and mind, and connects us to all other living things that breathe. The air you inhale with each breath has been breathed in and out by many others, past and present. Without turning my back on rationality and scientific method, I can say that I'm comfortable with the idea that breath represents the movement of spirit in the body and that we can become more aware of the spiritual self by paying attention to, observing, and meditating on the breath.

Realizing that essence and power are to be found less in the physical realm than the nonphysical has given me a richer understanding of

---

* Sanskrit *prana*, Hebrew *ruach*, Greek *pneuma*, Latin *spiritus*.

myself and the world around me. Although I have a unique body and a unique mind (if only because of my individual perceptions and memories), I feel that the spiritual essence of my being is the same as that of all beings. The more I maintain awareness of this feeling, the more connected I feel to others, and the more empathetic and compassionate I can be—qualities I consider essential to emotional wellness.

I chose the term *secular spirituality* in the title of this chapter to emphasize that it has nothing to do with any supernatural interpretations or explanations. Without believing in the supernatural, one can recognize aspects of human experience that are not accounted for in the materialistic view. (Even atheists and agnostics can embrace the interconnectedness of everything and the importance of living in harmony with nature and the universe.) In the following pages, I will tell you about strategies drawing on secular spirituality that I find complementary to the body- and mind-oriented methods I recommend. Some, like having flowers in your home and connecting with companion animals, may strike you as much more secular than spiritual. Others, like laughter therapy, might just as well be in the previous chapter. If you are still uncomfortable with the term *spirituality*, even when it is modified by *secular*, feel free to think of all of the strategies below as additional mind-oriented approaches to a better emotional life. On the other hand, if you are religious and connect with spirit primarily through religious faith and practice, consider the suggestions in this chapter as add-ons to enrich that experience.

Research on mind/body interactions and their potential usefulness in clinical medicine has long been hampered by the limitations of the biomedical model. Materialist philosophy insists that changes in physical systems must have physical causes; it does not allow for nonphysical causation of physical events. This bias stands in the way of greater acceptance of therapies like hypnosis and interactive guided imagery and has blinded doctors to the value of the placebo response (which I have long regarded as a physician's greatest ally). All this is now changing as a result of the new neuroscientific research I wrote about in chapter 4. Mind/body medicine is coming into its own, and more scientists are taking placebo responses seriously. But if it has taken this long to legitimize scientific inquiry into influences of the mind on the body and on health, imagine the obstacles to collecting evidence for the interplay of spirituality and health. There has been research on the healing effects of prayer and on correlations between religious affiliation and better health, but it does not shed light on the power of secular spirituality, and the findings are not central to the topic of this book. Whenever I can, I will cite studies to support the recommendations I'm about to give you; otherwise, I will back them up with my personal and professional experience.

Recall the words of sociologist Émile Durkheim: "Man cannot live without attachment to some object which transcends and survives him." I've suggested below ways to help you identify more closely with your nonphysical essence, to experience deeper connection to others, and to attach yourself to "objects" that transcend you.

CONNECT WITH NATURE

Although we are part of nature, nature is greater than us: infinite in its variety, fascinating in its ingenuity, able to inspire awe, reverence, and terror. We are creatures of nature and cannot enjoy optimum physical or emotional well-being if we have too little contact with it. Biologist E. O. Wilson coined the term *biophilia,* which means "love of life or living systems," to describe this innate human need. I believe it to be as real as our needs for food, sex, love, and community.

A few years ago, I got to go on a tour of one of our nuclear submarines. Of the many reasons that I would not be able to endure life on one of those vessels—for even a day or two, let alone months at a time—is the total disconnection from nature. Except for the crew (mostly very young men, chosen for duty after extensive psychological testing), I saw nothing natural on the sub—not even one living plant.

Sadly, that is not so different from the cold, sterile interiors of many office and apartment buildings. Human beings can survive in such places, but we cannot thrive in them.

I have been fortunate to live close to wilderness and spend ample time in relatively unspoiled natural settings for much of my life. But even if you live in the center of New York City or Tokyo or London, you can find ways to connect with nature in order to nourish your spiritual self. One way is to go to a park. New York's Central Park is magnificent; without it the city would be much less bearable. Growing up in a row house in Philadelphia, I was drawn to spend much time in equally wonderful Fairmount Park. Most cities have parks, public gardens, arboretums, and greenbelts. All you have to do is get to them and open yourself to the sights, sounds, and smells of nature they offer.

You can also bring bits of nature into your living space, even into a tiny apartment. House plants need some attention but give much in return. Get advice on species that will survive in the conditions of your home and select ones that you find attractive. And do try to keep fresh flowers around. For a minimal investment, you will have natural beauty at hand that will raise your spirits.

One of my hobbies is forcing* flowering bulbs for indoor bloom. In October, I chill tulip, narcissus, and hyacinth bulbs in the refrigerator. Then I pot them in late December, leave the pots in a protected spot against an outside wall, and keep them watered. Many people have no idea that these bulbs have within them fully formed "embryonic" leaves and flowers. Given water and minimal warmth, they come out of dormancy, sprout, and use the energy of sunlight to grow. When the flowering stalks show through the leaves, I bring the pots into my home, gradually exposing them to more light and warmth, and try not to be impatient for the show. I think of flowering bulbs as fireworks in slow

---

* An awful word: the bulbs are perfectly happy to be grown in this way, and despite what books say, they can be planted outdoors after they've flowered and will often bloom again in years following.

motion. (I love fireworks.) No matter how often I see these plants do their magic, I am always captivated by the beauty of the blooms and intoxicated by their fragrance. I get to enjoy spring in my own home while it is still winter outside, and my happiness soars as a result. I get further joy from sharing this gift with others by giving away containers of bulbs just about to pop.

Susan, sixty-eight, of Boynton Beach, Florida, describes her way of connecting with nature:

> I find that when I'm feeling blue, a visit to the nearby wetlands in my area of south Florida unfailingly lightens my mood and lifts my spirits. As soon as my feet hit the boardwalk that weaves its way through these places, my breathing gets slower and a smile comes to my face. My cares drop away as I walk. I love observing the wildlife that is living just feet away from the boardwalks. I find that being out in nature is my own best medicine.

In the interest of emotional well-being, I advise you to guard against nature deficit disorder by letting nature into your awareness as often as you can, any way you can. Watch the ever-changing shapes of clouds, admire trees, listen to the wind, look at the moon, at birds, at mountains. And when you do, be aware that you are part of nature, connected through it to something much larger than yourself that transcends and will survive you.

RELATE TO COMPANION ANIMALS

My family had several dogs when I was growing up. I bonded most with a female German shepherd we had for a few years when I was in junior high school and was devastated when we had to send her away; she needed more space and freedom than we could give her. I did not have another companion animal until I turned forty, when I was quite rootless and in the midst of a midlife crisis that included a rough patch of dysthymia. A longtime friend gave me a two-month-old female Rhodesian ridgeback as a birthday present. I told her that I couldn't take on a puppy; my life was too unsettled. She thrust the puppy in my arms and told me it would help get me settled. It did that and more, and dogs have been my companions ever since. I'm now on my third generation of ridgebacks, all raised from puppies, all true friends who have stuck with me through my worst moods, often lift me out of them, and often bring happiness into my life.

A great deal of scientific research confirms the benefits to health in general and emotional health in particular of living with companion animals—not only dogs but also cats, birds, and even reptiles and fish. Lynette A. Hart, PhD, a professor of veterinary medicine at the University of California, Davis, writes, "The comfort and contentment offered by animals is documented in a large number of studies with vulnerable people, including children, the elderly, and people with disability, disease, and loneliness." Remember comfort and contentment? Companion animals can bring more of both into your life. "Being around pets appears to feed the soul, promoting a sense of emotional connectedness and overall well-being," says another writer about pet therapy (or animal-assisted therapy), now a recognized treatment for depression and other mood disorders.

Let me tell you about some of the gifts I've received from my canine companions. They frequently remind me that spontaneous happiness is a real possibility, always available—by demonstrating it right in front of me. For example, they might pick up a bone or stick and race around wildly or dance with delight. They express ecstatic joy on my return after an absence, no matter whether of a week or an hour. They shower me with affection, even if I'm feeling low or disconnected. They encourage me to get outdoors and be physically active. They depend on me to take care of their needs and protect their health, preventing me from being overly focused on myself. If I'm more socially isolated than I should be, they keep me from feeling lonely. I think of them as family.

They touch my heart—and spirit. Often, I thank them for all of this, both with words and physical affection.

Having a companion animal is a responsibility. The decision to get one must be made thoughtfully, as should the choice of which one is right for you. The wrong animal can be a nuisance at the least or, worse, a major source of stress and trouble. If you are depressed as a result of loneliness, get stuck in depressive rumination because you are overly focused on yourself, or feel dispirited by lack of connection, consider the value of animal companionship. It can greatly enrich your life.

APPRECIATE ART AND BEAUTY

Beauty that people create can have the same power as natural beauty to take us out of negative thoughts and lift our spirits. Some years ago, I consulted with a Japanese society of energy healers who wanted to document the effects of their method by working with scientists. The method, called Johrei, sends energy through the hand to a recipient without physical contact. It was promoted by a spiritual teacher, Mokichi Okada (1882–1955), who founded one of modern Japan's many new religions. His teachings center on the existence of a spiritual world that coexists with the physical world and the need to receive its influence without interference. He advocated appreciation of art and beauty as one of the best ways to do that. Okada collected great art and established a world-famous art museum in the mountains above the coastal town of Atami; he also developed the Sangetsu school of flower arrangement. "It is important to develop and uplift human consciousness through beauty," he wrote. "For that purpose, I would like to encourage people to place flowers everywhere, as the best means of promoting the love of beauty." He also encouraged people to be around works of art.

I have visited Okada's museum and seen several Sangetsu exhibitions and enjoyed uplifted consciousness as a result. I experience the same feeling when I go to museums and stand in front of works of art and sculpture that move me or I discover aesthetically pleasing folk art and crafts at street fairs. I've brought back pottery and textiles that have caught my eye during my travels and placed them around my house. I have some fine old Bolivian weavings on my walls; I drink tea from a unique Japanese ceramic tea bowl that gladdens my spirit whenever I hold it, and I write at my desk under the benevolent gaze of a large carved statue of Ganesha, the elephant-headed Hindu deity known as the Lord of Success and Remover of Obstacles. My Ganesha is happily playing a drum. I got him when I visited Rajasthan a few years ago, and whenever I look at him, I feel happy.

Mary, fifty-one, a homemaker from Fort Mill, South Carolina, writes:

> My husband and I relocated from Massachusetts to South Carolina in 2004. A month before, I put my mother in a nursing home because she had Alzheimer's. Needless to say I felt terrible and guilty for moving away. I made trips to Massachusetts every six to eight weeks to visit my mother. Leaving became harder and harder and I would get very depressed and cry all the way back. After about a year of this, I decided to spend the afternoons before I planned to leave my mother at either the Museum of Fine Arts or one of the other museums in Boston. Taking the time to look at all the beauty art provides calmed me right down, and even though I was still sad to leave, walking around all that enduring art changed my perspective and I stopped being depressed.

Of course, beauty is a matter of personal taste (even when it comes to flowers). I wouldn't presume to tell you what kind of art or crafts you should appreciate, but as part of the secular spiritual approach to emotional wellness, I suggest that you take time to expose yourself to art and beauty in various forms and expressions and keep objects that you find beautiful in your living space.

Try Putting Others First

If you live with a dog or cat, you sometimes have to put its interests and needs ahead of your own. If you live with a spouse, children, or an aging parent, you often have to subordinate your needs to theirs. When situations force us to do this, it is easy to resent the demands on our attention and time, but putting others first is a practice commonly recommended to stimulate self-development and spiritual growth. It turns out also to be an effective strategy to enhance emotional wellness. In addition to reducing social isolation, it helps decrease the self-focus that favors depressive rumination, and it can lead to greater empathy and compassion.

We've been told that goodness is its own reward. In fact, doing good for others brings a very tangible reward in the form of benefits to physical and mental health. In his 2001 book, *The Healing Power of Doing Good,* the former Peace Corps volunteer and community action lawyer Allan Luks introduced the term "helper's high" to describe the rush of good feelings that people get when they help others. He proposed that it was an endorphin-mediated state analogous to the well-known "runner's high." Since then, neuroscientists have demonstrated that helping others activates the same centers in the brain involved in dopamine-mediated pleasure responses to food and sex. In one study, these pleasure centers lit up when participants simply thought about giving money to a charity.

From a study of more than three thousand volunteers, Luks concluded that regular helpers are ten times more likely to be in good health than people who don't volunteer. One sociologist and happiness expert, Christine L. Carter, PhD, writes that "giving help to others protects overall health twice as much as aspirin protects against heart disease." She goes on to say:

> People fifty-five and older who volunteer for two or more organizations have an impressive 44 percent lower likelihood of dying—and that's after sifting out every other contributing factor, including

physical health, exercise, gender, habits like smoking, marital status, and many more. This is a stronger effect than exercising four times a week or going to church; it means that volunteering is nearly as beneficial to our health as quitting smoking!

Helpers are also less likely to be depressed and more likely to be happy. One of the findings of the landmark Social Capital Community Benchmark Survey of almost thirty thousand Americans, published in 2000, was that those who give contributions of time or money are 42 percent more likely to be happy than those who don't give. That's why I recommend that you try putting others first. There are many ways to do so, both in thought and action. You could join the Peace Corps or volunteer for relief work in a disaster area, but I believe you can get similar emotional benefits just by being more aware of the suffering of others and giving some of your time and energy to alleviating it. You can perform acts of altruism, as ordinary as being more courteous when you're behind the wheel of your car. You can resolve to be kinder in your dealings with others. It all works. Kindness and generosity toward others can actually make you happier.

If you behave altruistically in order to get a helper's high, improve your health, or be happy, are you really being altruistic? Is charity "really self-interest masquerading under the form of altruism," in the words of Anthony de Mello, a Jesuit priest? Does it matter? The Dalai Lama uses the term *selfish altruism* without any pejorative sense. And Corinthians 9:7 advises that "God loveth a cheerful giver," which to me indicates that it's also fine in the Christian faith to become happy by giving. Everybody wins.

When I consider the ways that I've tried to give to others and what I've received in return, I see that some forms of giving have made me happier than others. I don't get much of a helper's high from writing year-end checks to charities and deserving organizations, but I get great ones from helping people one-on-one, especially through teaching and sharing my knowledge. I give that away for free as much as I do for pay, and freely giving it makes me feel very good. In 2005 I was able to create a private foundation funded mostly by donating all of my after-tax profits from royalties on sales of retail products licensed by Weil Lifestyle, LLC. To date, it has given more than $2 million in grants to nonprofit institutions in the medical sciences to advance the field of integrative medicine. As a member of the board of directors, I take great pleasure in making these grants and following the beneficial effects they produce. Over the years, friends involved with family foundations have told me of the happiness they enjoy from being philanthropic. I now understand that.

Terry, sixty-seven, of Monroe, Washington has this to say:

> You asked about the "helper's high"—I had never thought about it that way before, but I must say, I experience it now on a regular basis! Not only am I a grandma of two-year-old natural triplets that I help with every day, I'm also a CASA [Court Appointed Special Advocates] volunteer, carrying five cases at the moment. Giving is truly a gift FROM me and TO me. Helping raise my grandbabies is such a blessing, and being an advocate for abused/neglected kids fills my heart each day with more joy than I'm able to explain. Giving of myself is truly the best high of them all!!

The only times I don't feel happy when I help others are when I become blasé about it, do too much of it, or do it out of a sense of obligation rather than generosity. It is important to remember to take care of yourself. Helpers can overextend themselves, become depleted as a result, and burn out. Some people get into this fix because they consider it selfish to attend to their own needs when the needs of those they care for are so great. If you find yourself thinking that way, take a lesson from your heart. The first thing your heart does with the oxygen-rich blood it receives from the lungs is to nourish itself through the coronary arteries. It does so before it sends any to the rest of the body. If it did not take care of itself, it would not be able to give you a lifetime of service. Selfish altruism? Whatever you call it, putting others first—whether to help them, increase your happiness, or both—does not mean neglecting your own needs.

LEARN EMPATHY AND COMPASSION

Empathy is the ability to feel what others feel, to know another person's experience because you can connect it with your own. Compassion is understanding what others feel and using that understanding to respond to them with love and kindness. We think of empathy and compassion as virtues, but they are also learnable skills that can bring greater happiness into your life and improve all of your relationships. You can sign up today for various forms of empathy training, not just Buddhist meditation classes but secular business courses designed to make you a better negotiator or manager. In the business world, empathy is held in high regard for the simple reason that people who are most empathetic tend to be most successful.

Empathy and compassion favor communication and social bonding. They strengthen community and mitigate interpersonal strife and violence. To hurt or kill another human being, one must first define that person as "other"—different from you in some essential way. Empathy prevents that.

Compassion meditation is a Buddhist practice that includes thinking about the suffering of others and generating positive feelings, first toward loved ones and eventually toward all people, wishing them well-being, happiness, and freedom from suffering. Doing this is good for us as well as others. The Dalai Lama has said that

> compassion and affection help the brain to function more smoothly. Secondarily, compassion gives us inner strength; it gives us self-confidence and that reduces fear, which, in turn, keeps our mind calm. Therefore, compassion has two functions: it causes our brain to

function better and it brings inner strength. These, then, are the causes of happiness.

In his brain-imaging studies, Richard Davidson and colleagues have documented changes in the brains of both Tibetan monks and laypersons trained in compassion meditation. They found significant activity in the insula, a brain region that mediates bodily representations of emotion, as well as in the right temporoparietal junction, which appears to be involved in detecting the emotional states of others and in processing empathy. In one ingenious study, subjects (all trained meditators) were placed in the fMRI (functional magnetic resonance imaging) scanner and asked to begin compassion meditation or refrain from it. They were then exposed to negative, positive, and neutral human sounds — a woman crying out in distress, a baby laughing, and background restaurant noise. When the subjects were generating compassion, their empathic response to the positive and negative vocalizations was much greater, as indicated by increased activity of the two brain regions. Furthermore, the magnitude of activation correlated with the intensity of the meditation as reported by the subjects.

In his excellent book *The Compassionate Mind,* psychologist Paul Gilbert, who heads the Mental Health Research Unit at the University of Derby (UK), points out that mindfulness and compassion are closely related; he writes that the essence of compassion is being *here, now, with another* — not *there, then, with your thoughts.* He gives a number of exercises to develop these skills, one of them being the creation of a compassionate mental image to use as an object of meditative practice or to focus on whenever you feel stressed or sad. Gilbert recommends creating your own image from scratch, putting thought into whether you want it to be old or young, male or female, human or nonhuman. Whatever form you choose, it should be wise, strong, kind, warm, nurturing, and nonjudgmental, and desirous of your well-being and happiness.

Learning empathy and compassion contribute to emotional wellness by promoting spiritual growth. These skills allow you to identify with others on a deep level, lessening isolation and loneliness. They offer protection from depression and greater possibilities for experiencing spontaneous happiness.

Practice Forgiveness

Philosophers and saints commonly teach that forgiveness is one key to happiness. The reason, they say, is that it calms the mind and spirit and neutralizes resentment. Resentment fuels one of the most toxic forms of depressive rumination: running thought loops over and over about past hurts. "He robbed me." "I loved her, and she betrayed me." "Why does he treat me like that?" "They stole my idea." Formulations of this sort undermine emotional health. Get rid of them if you want more spontaneous happiness in your life.

To *forgive* is "to give something up or let something go"— specifically the desire to punish or take revenge on one who has hurt or wronged you. You do it for yourself, not for another. (Never mind Oscar Wilde's advice to "always forgive your enemies—nothing annoys them so much.") In practicing forgiveness, you acknowledge your connection and identity with other beings and in so doing improve spiritual well-being and decrease loneliness. Learning empathy and compassion makes it easier to forgive, because those skills allow you to see things from others' viewpoints, feel what they feel, and understand why they may have wronged you.

Research shows that those who forgive enjoy better social interactions in general and become more altruistic over time. Improvements in both physical and emotional well-being follow acts of forgiving, and a 2009 study documents an inverse correlation between forgiveness and depression. Merely remembering occasions when you forgave can bring you closer to other people. And we even know something about the neurological mechanisms involved, such as activation of the right temporoparietal junction, the same brain region associated with empathy and the capacity to understand the beliefs and perspectives of others.

If forgiving is so good for us, why can it be so hard to do? When I find it difficult to forgive, it is mostly because I don't want to exonerate the other person, don't want to make his or her offensive actions all right. If the same feeling gets in your way, it might help to know that scholarly definitions of forgiveness often specify that it does not condone the offensive behavior, minimize its gravity, or imply that the perpetrator was not responsible for the act. I try to remind myself that for me, forgiveness means that those who wronged me will have to deal with the consequences of their actions on their own, independent of my reactions to them. When I'm totally honest with myself, I have to admit that my reluctance to forgive might also have an element of satisfaction in nursing the emotional hurt, just as it can be satisfying to attend obsessively to a physical wound. Bringing that into full awareness helps me let it go.

I advise you to *practice* forgiveness, because it is a process that requires conscious effort and ongoing commitment. If you feel you need help with this, you can try various interventions, such as a six-hour "empathy-oriented forgiveness seminar," in which you will be asked to describe past incidents of being wronged or hurt and then consider different strategies for coping with your feelings. Participants are also encouraged to try to understand the thoughts and feelings of persons who acted offensively as well as to think about their own feelings when they have been forgiven by someone else.

Dr. Frederic Luskin, who directs the Stanford Forgiveness Project at Stanford University, has documented the effectiveness of such training, which he presents in books, audio and video programs, and online courses (www.learningtoforgive.com). He has worked with mediators and others interested in conflict resolution, and some of his trainees are using his methods to help bring peace to conflict-torn areas of the world. Luskin's doctoral dissertation was on the spiritual quality of forgiveness. He wrote, "For me it was a limitation that we were so bound from connecting the material, tangible, and measurable world to spiritual questions and pursuits." I agree. That's why I've put this information on the emotional rewards of forgiveness under the heading of secular spirituality.

Here is an account of the power of forgiveness from Marcia, fifty-three, an administrative assistant in Katy, Texas:

> When I was two years old, my mother remarried. She and my stepfather were married for eight years. This man was abusive, physically and verbally, and I received a lot of it. Even though they divorced when I was ten, I was angry for decades. The abuse affected every aspect of my life. I even married a man much like my stepfather when I was twenty-one but divorced a year later. I would spend sleepless nights wishing my stepfather dead and blaming him for everything that had gone wrong in my life.
>
> When I was forty-five, I saw him again, at my mother's home. He was in town getting chemo treatments for cancer and had been invited to a family get-together. He didn't even recognize me! I was so incredibly angry at all that he had put me through, how he had ruined my life, and now he didn't even remember all that he had done or even who I was. Incredible! I contemplated this situation for a couple of hours at my mother's get-together, had a drink or two, then walked up to him, kissed him on the cheek, and told him, "You know, I really loved you once," and in my heart I forgave him for all the abusive years.
>
> Next day, I woke up free from all the anger, free from the guilt, free from the shame. I haven't had a moment's anguish from that man's actions again. I feel lighter, stronger, more confident. I can't believe that I let so much of my life be lived under a dark cloud when all I had to do was forgive, and the cloud was gone.

The bottom line: We now have scientific evidence to support the idea—advanced over centuries—that forgiving can make you feel better.

SMILE AND LAUGH

When it comes to expressing positive emotion, the common belief is that cause and effect work in one direction. First comes a happy feeling. That's followed by a smile or maybe a laugh. Then, when the feeling runs its natural course, the outward expression stops. The one-way journey from *feeling* to *showing* is over.

The facial-feedback hypothesis of emotional expression is an alternative explanation. It holds that physically expressing an emotion sends a biochemical signal from the facial muscles that "loops" back to the brain, in much the same way that sound coming from a speaker can be picked up by a microphone and sent back through the speaker as amplified feedback. Charles Darwin was among the first scientists to put forth this idea, stating that "the free expression by outward signs of an emotion intensifies it. On the other hand, the repression, as far as this is possible, of all outward signs softens our emotions.... Even the simulation of an emotion tends to arouse it in our minds."

The best way to test this theory is to simulate the muscular contractions of a facial expression and see if this changes the subject's emotional state. A 1988 study by researchers at Universität Mannheim, Federal Republic of Germany, did just that. Participants were told to hold a pen in their mouths in one of two ways—in their lips, which activated the *orbicularis oris* muscle, used in frowning; or in their teeth, which employed the *zygomatic major* or *risorius* muscle, used in smiling. A control group simply held the pen in their hands. Then the three groups were shown a cartoon, and told to evaluate how funny they found it.

Members of the "teeth" group reported finding the cartoon significantly more amusing than did those in the "lips" or control group. Further, the study was carefully designed to prevent any "cognitive interpretation of the facial action"—in other words, unlike previous studies that instructed participants to fake a smile or frown, this one gave them no clues whatsoever as to what kinds of emotions they might be expected to feel.

This and similar studies demonstrate clearly that emotions stimulate physical expressions, *and* physical expressions stimulate emotions. That gives scientific support to such corny song lyrics as "Smile and the whole world smiles with you!" It also makes me even more uneasy about the widespread use of injections of onabotulinumtoxinA (Botox) to remove wrinkles by paralyzing facial muscles; that treatment may actually inhibit the ability to feel emotion.

The facial-feedback mechanism that works individually also works on a group level. When we see or hear people laugh, we tend to laugh ourselves, which makes them laugh more, and so on. This means that a group of laughing people constitutes a powerful collection of *internal* and *external* feedback loops of positive emotion, making laughing together one of life's greatest pleasures. Watching funny movies with friends and attending comic performances are informal ways to enjoy these wonderful, complex, social webs of good feeling, but a relatively new practice known as laughter yoga (or laughter therapy) creates such situations specifically and intentionally. Begun by Dr. Madan Kataria, a physician from Mumbai, India, the first laughter club convened in March of 1995 with a handful of people. Now, according to the official laughter yoga website, there are more than six thousand Social Laughter Clubs in sixty countries. I've met Dr. Kataria and had the pleasure of laughing with him. He knew that laughter was the best medicine and wondered how to get people to do more of it. His great discovery was that when people in groups simulate laughter, it rapidly becomes real.

Real laughter involves activity of the involuntary nervous system: tearing of the eyes, spasms of the diaphragm, and flushing of the face. It gets out of control and can leave you doubled up on the floor. And it feels so good at the time and afterward. In the magnitude and immediacy of its mood-boosting effect, it puts the most powerful antidepressant drugs to shame.

The method used in laughter clubs is straightforward. After brief physical exercises and breathing exercises under the direction of a trained leader, people simulate laughter with vigorous ha-ha's and ho-ho's. In the group setting, this fake laughter quickly becomes real and contagious and may continue for a half hour or more. The end result is joy and good fellowship. And the joy lingers; regular participation in laughter clubs has been shown to improve long-term emotional and physical health in a variety of ways, including a significant lowering of the stress hormone cortisol.

If you want to take part in a laughter club, the good news is that these groups are, like laughter itself, free and easy: there are no membership fees, no forms to fill out, no complications. The clubs are run by trained volunteers. Laughter clubs are nonpolitical, nonreligious, and nonprofit. They are overseen by Laughter Clubs International in India, and Laughter Yoga International in other countries. For more information, go to www.laughteryoga.org.

If the formalized practice of laughter yoga doesn't appeal to you, simply understand—as Darwin noted—that expressing emotion is a key component of *feeling* emotion. Many people laugh only a little, or quietly, as if they feel to laugh long and loudly is undignified, an unacceptable behavior. This may be a product of culture. Japanese often cover their mouths when laughing, as if to conceal it. Conversely, I have known Brazilians who habitually throw the head back and roar with laughter, sometimes even collapsing as a group into a giggling, exhausted heap. I respect both cultures, but here I think the Brazilians have the better idea.

If you allow yourself only half smiles and occasional guffaws, try opening up and letting go the next time you feel the urge. You may find yourself at the center of your own, spontaneously generated laughter club and leave everyone in your world—including you—happier for having done so.

CULTIVATE SILENCE

Essays on the value of silence, and sayings like "Silence is golden," advise us not to talk so much. I have little patience with people who can't keep quiet, and I have discovered the way that I best acquire knowledge and useful information is to listen rather than talk. But in recommending that you cultivate silence, I'm asking you to limit what you hear more than what you say. I have already discussed the adverse impact on our moods of the noise of modern life. I believe that making an effort to experience silence regularly, even if briefly, helps counteract that and supports our well-being—physical, mental, and spiritual.

It may take serious effort. Quiet times and places are hard to find—so hard, in fact, that I wonder if we are afraid of silence. "Why?" asks the English writer and literary critic Susan Hill. "Are we afraid of what we will discover when we come face-to-face with ourselves there? Perhaps there will be nothing but a great void, nothing within us, and nothing outside of us either. Terrifying. Let's drown our fears with some noise, quickly." I once sat in an anechoic chamber, a room insulated against all sound, used in acoustics research; the unnatural silence in it was almost palpable, and after a few minutes I found it oppressive. But I welcome natural silence, especially when I go from a noisy environment into a quiet one; the contrast totally refreshes me, much as a long, cool drink of water does when I am hot and thirsty. If silence scares you, dip into it briefly but often to become tolerant to it and lose any fear of it you may have.

I agree with Susan Hill that "silence is a rich and fertile soil in which many things grow and flourish, not least an awareness of everything outside oneself and apart from oneself, as well, paradoxically, as everything within." That's why I put cultivation of silence under the heading of secular spirituality. It fosters mindfulness and all the mental and emotional benefits of bringing full conscious awareness to the present moment.

If you search them out, you can discover oases of relative quiet in big cities: in libraries and reading rooms, museums, houses of worship, parks, and gardens. Most of the hospitals I've worked in have had meditation rooms, and I've used them to escape from all the stress-inducing sounds on the wards and in the corridors, even if only for a few minutes here and there. I also take advantage of quiet times of day and night, getting up just before dawn, when most of the world around me is not yet stirring. I find it easiest to meditate then, and afterward I like to go on walks with my dogs, watch the sun rise, and enjoy the streets around my home before there is any traffic. The evening dusk can be almost as quiet, and I welcome nighttime silence. Should I happen to find myself awake in the middle of the night, instead of trying to go back to sleep, I soak up the silence, feel grateful for it, and focus on my breathing until I drift off.

Get better at managing the electronic sounds in your environment, turning off televisions and radios unless there are programs that interest you, silencing ringers and beepers, switching cell phones to vibrate. Avoid noisy people and places. Cultivate silence in your life and let it heal and refresh you whenever you encounter it.

CHOOSE THE RIGHT COMPANY

The term *infectious happiness* suggests that emotions can spread from person to person by contact, like contagious diseases. I'm sure you know people in whose company you feel more positive and optimistic and others who bring you down. We now have scientific evidence for emotional contagion that not only describes and quantifies the ways communicable moods spread through social networks but also makes a strong case for choosing right company. For example, if you have a happy friend who lives within a mile of you, your chance of happiness increases by 25 percent.

That is one finding of a study published in the *British Medical Journal* in 2008 that analyzed data on 4,739 people who were followed from 1983 to 2003 in the Framingham Heart Study. Others are that live-in partners who become happy raise the likelihood of their partners' happiness by 8 percent, that siblings who live close by can boost your happiness by 14 percent, neighbors by 34 percent. Close proximity facilities the spread of infectious happiness. You have a greater chance—42 percent greater—of being happy if a friend who lives less than half a mile away becomes happy. That effect then declines with greater distance, eventually becoming insignificant. The authors of the study, a social scientist from Harvard Medical School and a political scientist at the University of California, San Diego, concluded that "changes in individual happiness can ripple through social networks and generate large-scale structure in the network, giving rise to clusters of happy...people."

Other analyses of the same data show that negative emotions are just as transmissible as positive ones. The more contact you have with people who are discontented, the more likely you are to become discontented. The same is true of depression. Clinical psychologist Michael Yapko published a book in 2009 titled *Depression Is Contagious: How the Most Common Mood Disorder Is Spreading Around the World and How to Stop It.* He identifies bad relationships as the core problem and urges readers to develop the social skills necessary to build good ones.

I like to think that human beings "resonate" with one another in the dimension of spirit, analogous to the way a vibrating tuning fork induces another one near it to vibrate at the same rate. Whatever the mechanism, there is no question that the people you choose to associate with can raise or lower your spirits, make you happy or sad, calm or anxious, comfortable or uncomfortable. Therefore I ask you to take care to choose the right company.

FEEL AND EXPRESS GRATITUDE

We have strong evidence of the power of gratitude to boost mood. You can read about the studies in a recent book: *Thanks! How Practicing Gratitude Can Make You Happier* by Robert A. Emmons, professor of psychology at the University of California, Davis, and editor in chief of the *Journal of Positive Psychology.* "Practicing gratitude?" You are not likely to have heard of it, because it is new. The most significant finding to date is that regularly practicing grateful thinking can move your emotional set point for happiness by as much as 25 percent in the right direction. That's big news, because it challenges the conventional assumption that our emotional set point is set for life. Until the practice of gratitude got going, most psychologists believed that an individual's capacity to experience happiness was fixed at birth—a product of genetics and brain structure that cannot be influenced by experience, environment, or conscious effort. Now it appears that, as with many human traits, an interaction of inherited and noninherited factors governs where on the spectrum of emotions we tend to spend most time.

From the research data that I have reviewed, I consider expressing gratitude to be one of the very best strategies to enhance emotional well-being, right up there with fish oil, physical activity, and managing negative thoughts. Like forgiveness, gratitude can be cultivated.

To be grateful is to acknowledge receipt of something of value—a gift, a favor, a blessing—to feel thankful for it and be inclined to give kindness in return. *Gratitude* comes from Latin *gratus,* meaning "grateful." To get something gratis, from the Latin *gratia,* meaning "favor," is to get it free, without expectation of payment. Another word of the same origin is *grace,* defined in theology as the "freely given, unmerited favor and love of god" and sometimes combined redundantly with yet another closely related word in the phrase *gratuitous grace,* meaning grace freely given by god to particular individuals without regard to their morality or behavior.

Most of us are familiar with the act of saying grace before meals as an expression of thankfulness for food received. Our family did not do so when I was growing up, and I was uncomfortable when I first shared meals with people who did, because it seemed to be a religious ritual that required belief in a deity. In my travels through the counterculture of America in the late 1960s and early 1970s, I got in the habit of holding hands with people around dinner tables, sometimes sharing a few moments of silent gratitude for the food and company, sometimes chanting an *aum* or singing a song. Then, on frequent trips to Japan, I became familiar with the custom of beginning meals by placing the palms together in front of the heart and saying aloud *itadakimasu,* often translated as "bon appétit," but really meaning "I humbly receive." I have adopted it as a secular form of saying grace, of expressing gratitude for food on the table.

Emmons conceives of gratitude in two stages:

> First, gratitude is acknowledgment of goodness in one's own life. In gratitude we say yes to life. We affirm that all things taken together, life is good and has elements that make it worth living. The acknowledgment that we have received something gratifies us, either by its presence or by the effort the giver went to in choosing it. Second, gratitude is recognizing that the source(s) of this goodness lie at least partially outside the self. The object of gratitude is other-directed; one can be grateful to other people, to God, to animals, but never to oneself.... Thanks are directed outward to the giver of gifts.

I would add that feeling grateful and expressing gratitude are distinct. To get maximum emotional reward, you will want to do both. You can remind yourself to feel grateful; you may have to learn and try out different ways of expressing it. It is much easier to get better at this than at forgiving, because there are no bad feelings to get in the way, nothing to get over or give up. The only impediment is the common tendency to take for granted the gifts and blessings we receive.

What do you have to be grateful for? How about being alive for starters? Or enjoying good health? Or being able to put food on your table, food of better quality and greater variety than people have ever had? It is a time of relative peace. You have shelter, warmth in winter, material comforts beyond the imaginings of our ancestors. The sun freely gives you light, warmth, and the energy that makes your food. If you happen to watch the sun rise, that might be a good occasion to feel grateful for its gifts. I find that if I don't create such occasions, I forget to feel grateful. It's just so easy to take it all for granted. And having a Thanksgiving feast once a year is not going to move your set point for happiness.

The method used most frequently in research on the effects of practicing gratitude is the Gratitude Journal. Subjects are asked to dedicate a notebook to this, to make mental notes throughout the day about things to be grateful for, and to enter them in the book at some regular time, such as bedtime.

Jennifer, forty-one, of Plano, Texas, who suffers from multiple sclerosis, reports:

> A gratitude journal has changed the way I think and how I react to things. I look for the positives and find it easier to dismiss negative thoughts. I'm currently going through a five-day IV steroid treatment for my MS and just wrote in my journal that I'm grateful for the medication. I'm grateful for the nurse who comes every day. I'm grateful that I can work while having this treatment that's going to make me stronger and more productive. Those thoughts outweigh the fact that my arm hurts, that I haven't been sleeping well and at times I'm a little cranky. The journal puts things in perspective that could have gotten lost if I wallowed in the negatives, and I used to be pretty good at wallowing. I think it's made me happier, certainly easier to be around.

Another method is the Gratitude Visit, which I described in chapter 6 as one of the interventions of positive psychology: writing a letter of appreciation to someone who has had a beneficial influence on you, then meeting that person and reading the letter to him or her face-to-face.

I have not used either of these techniques, but I do try to take a few moments of my morning meditation to feel and silently give thanks for all that I have to be grateful for. As a result of doing this for a number of years, I find myself more often making mental notes of things to be grateful for throughout the day: flowers that have opened in or around my home, the unconditional love I feel from my dogs, a glorious sunset, rain in the desert, the gift of friendship, the resilience of my body.

The point of practicing both feeling and expressing gratitude is to change your perspective. "Gratitude is an attitude" may be a platitude, but it happens to be true: by becoming aware of what you have to be grateful for, you will find more and more to be grateful for. You will become less pessimistic and more optimistic, learn to see the glass as half full rather than half empty. (A friend tells me his extremely anxious and pessimistic mother not only sees the glass as half empty but thinks "it could tip over at any moment, spill on the floor, and break.") I believe this change in attitude and perspective gets the emotional set point unstuck and opens us to greater happiness.

Over the years, many writers, poets, philosophers, and teachers have penned words about gratitude. My favorite quote—short and to the point—is from English poet, painter, and printmaker William Blake (1757–1827): "The thankful receiver bears a plentiful harvest." Spontaneous happiness can be a major part of that harvest.

A SUMMARY OF SECULAR SPIRITUAL APPROACHES TO EMOTIONAL WELL-BEING

- Insufficient contact with nature predisposes us to depression. Find ways to connect with nature. Take advantage of city parks. Bring natural beauty into your living space.
- If you are sad as a result of feeling lonely or lack social connection, consider bringing a companion animal into your life. Be sure to think first about the responsibility of caring for an animal and the importance of choosing one that is right for you and your situation. The emotional rewards of animal companionship are great.
- Expose yourself to art and beauty. Doing so can get you out of negative moods and uplift your spirit. Keep fresh flowers in your home and surround yourself with beautiful objects.

- Without neglecting your own needs, try putting others first more of the time. Lend a helping hand—by volunteering, doing service work, or just doing favors for people. You will get a helper's high in return and become a happier person over time.
- Learn to be more empathetic and compassionate. By feeling and understanding what others feel, you will develop better relationships and increase your emotional well-being.
- Practice forgiveness as a way of letting go of negative thoughts and emotions that may be preventing you from enjoying optimum emotional health. Remember that forgiving is for you, not for anyone else.
- Laugh! Spend more time with people you can laugh with. Try going to a laughter group.
- Seek out places and times that provide silence. Silence refreshes the spirit, reduces anxiety, and makes it easier to be mindful.
- Spend more time with people who are optimistic, positive, and happy, less with people who are pessimistic, anxious, or depressed. Emotions are contagious.
- Remind yourself to feel grateful for all that you have and learn to express gratitude frequently. This is the easiest and best way to move your emotional set point toward greater happiness and positivity.

PART THREE

PUTTING IT ALL TOGETHER

8

An 8-Week Program for Optimum Emotional Well-Being

Y ou now understand that the foundation of emotional wellness is contentment, serenity, and comfort. It is normal for moods to vary. It is normal to experience both negative and positive emotions as appropriate responses to life events, but your ups and downs should balance each other, and you should have the resilience to come back to your center. You should not get emotionally stuck. Nor should your moods undermine your physical health, interfere with your sleep or work, damage your relationships, or limit you from engaging fully with life. If you feel you have too little spontaneous happiness, know that you can make changes to let more of it in.

The suggestions and strategies I have given you for optimizing emotional well-being derive from an integrative model of mental health. They address all factors that affect your moods. Selecting the ones best suited to your individual needs and working with them diligently will be more effective than simply relying on medications that target brain chemistry. I have explained the rationale for these recommendations and the scientific data that support them. It is now up to you to implement them.

To help you with that, I have organized the prescriptive information in chapters 5, 6, and 7 into an eight-week program. In each week, I will give you one or more assignments. (In some cases, I will ask you to try out several options to find what works best for you.) Of course, some of the assignments—such as changing your diet, exploring cognitive behavioral therapy, and regularly expressing gratitude—require long-term commitment. But you can easily take the first steps in the course of a week, and I promise you that after two months, when you "graduate," you will enjoy enhanced emotional well-being.

Feel free to proceed through the program at your own pace, taking as much time as you need with the assignments. If you want to spend two weeks instead of one with each section, by all means do so. And be patient with yourself: in my experience, it takes at least eight weeks to realize the effects of lifestyle changes on health, both physical and emotional.

Week 1: Getting Started

In order to start a journey, you need to know where you are and where you want to go. Your assignments this week are to assess your present state of health, review your lifestyle, and set goals. I'm going to ask you a series of questions. Write the answers down. I'll review them with you in order to identify your most pressing needs.

Questions About Your General Health

- Do you have any illnesses?
- Do you have any symptoms that concern you?
- Are you taking any prescribed or over-the-counter medications?
- Are you regularly taking any dietary supplements or herbal remedies?
- When did you last have a complete medical examination with blood work? Was anything abnormal?
- Are there any illnesses that run in your family?
- On a scale from 1 to 10, with 1 being "very unhealthy" and 10 being "very healthy," rate your present state of health.

Questions About Your Emotional Health

- Have you ever been diagnosed with a mood disorder?
- Have you ever consulted a mental health professional?
- Have you ever suffered from depression or anxiety?
- Do mental health issues run in your family?
- Do you tend to be pessimistic or optimistic?
- In general, on a scale from 1 to 10, with 1 being "very sad" and 10 being "very happy," where is your emotional set point?
- What do you think would make you happier?
- Do you recover quickly from emotional setbacks?
- Do you experience serenity in your life? How much of the time are you content? Comfortable?

Questions About Your Lifestyle

- Do you think you eat a healthy diet?
- Do you enjoy eating?
- How much of what you eat is refined, processed, and manufactured food?
- How much caffeine do you consume? In what forms?
- Have you ever been a smoker? Or used other forms of tobacco?
- Do you drink alcohol? If so, what kinds, how much, how often, and in what circumstances?
- Do you use any recreational drugs?
- Do you get regular physical activity? What kind? How much and how often? What keeps you from being more active?
- How well do you sleep?
- Rate your level of stress on a scale from 1 to 5, with 1 being "no stress at all" and 5 being "very stressed." How does stress affect you? How do you manage it?
- What is the main source of stress in your life?
- What do you do to relax?
- What do you do for fun?
- Do you enjoy your work?

Personal Questions

- Are your relationships satisfactory?
- Do you feel you get enough emotional nurturing from social interaction? Enough social support?
- Do you have good friends?
- Do you get stuck in thought patterns that make you depressed or anxious?
- How do you get yourself out of negative moods?
- How difficult is it for you to limit your time on the Internet, e-mail, and cell phones?

- How many happy friends and relatives do you have? Do they live near you? Do you see them often? Are your housemates and neighbors happy?
- Are you religious? Do you practice? Do you attend religious services?
- Is spirituality of interest to you? Where in your life do you experience spirituality?
- How often do you connect with nature?
- Do you have a companion animal?
- Are you a forgiving person?
- Are you grateful? Do you express gratitude?
- How easily and often do you laugh?

Let's go over your answers.

If you have health concerns or any symptoms that might indicate underlying disease, please get a medical checkup before you start this program. Especially, make sure that you do not have any hormonal imbalances or disorders of immunity that might be affecting your moods.

If you feel you are not in optimum health, I want you to know that many of the recommendations I will give you, such as the Anti-Inflammatory Diet (see Appendix A) and regular physical activity, are key elements of a lifestyle that favors overall wellness and longevity. You will feel better, physically as well as emotionally, if you follow them.

If you have a history of major depression or bipolar disorder, do not use this program as a substitute for medication or professional mental health care. It can be of great help to you along with conventional treatment, and I suggest that you discuss it with your mental health care provider. Ask him or her to monitor your progress.

Next, look over your answers to the questions about your lifestyle. Where are you strong? Where weak? Maybe you eat well but don't exercise. Stress could be your main problem, or lack of sleep. Maybe you are lonely and isolated. Or you might enjoy good physical health and have good habits of eating and activity but be subject to negative thoughts that make you sad or anxious. Or you may never have thought about spirituality and its influence on your moods and outlook.

Write down the lifestyle areas in which you are weakest. As you move ahead through the program in the coming days and weeks, pay particular attention to the elements that address them, and promise yourself that by the end of Week 8 you will have made substantial improvements in all of them.

Now think about what you most need from this program. Do you want help with depression? If so, you should prioritize recommendations about diet, dietary supplements, physical activity, mental nutrition, and social interaction. Do you need to control anxiety? If so, pay special attention to my suggestions about caffeine, physical activity, sleep, the 4-7-8 breath, noise, and information overload. In Week 4, I'll ask you to start experimenting with the natural remedies I recommend for depression and anxiety.

Do you want greater emotional resilience and balance? If so, use the program to create a more balanced lifestyle by eating well every day, spending time in nature, giving equal attention to work and play, improving sleep, and being physically active. Find a form of meditation that suits you and practice it. Do you want more contentment, comfort, and serenity? Meditation practice can bring those, as will all of the weekly recommendations under the heading "Caring for Your Spirit."

Are you generally free from depression but nonetheless want to move your emotional set point toward greater positivity? If so, work with the exercises of positive psychology starting in Week 4 and give special attention to feeling and expressing gratitude.

Do you want more spontaneous happiness in your life? Open yourself to it by completing all the weekly assignments. By doing so, you will be fine-tuning your lifestyle to create optimum emotional well-being.

Finally, write down your primary goal for this journey. Also write down any secondary goals. Read this over as you start each week of the program. At the end of Week 8, I will ask you to assess your progress toward these goals and think about the work you need to do in following weeks to solidify the changes you have made and go farther.

Week 2: First Things First

This week, you'll take your first big steps toward your goal by addressing any outstanding health issues, beginning to modify your diet, starting on the recommended supplements, attending to your physical activity, and familiarizing yourself with the breathing technique that will become a powerful tool over the next few weeks.

Caring for Your Body

- If you have not had a complete medical checkup in the past five years, schedule one. Find out if you are due for any diagnostic or screening tests. Give blood samples for comprehensive tests; make sure they include determination of thyroid function and your level of 25-hydroxy-vitamin D. (If you've never had your vitamin D level measured, get that done even if you do not need a complete physical exam.)
- Review the information on pages 103 to 104 about the mood-altering effects of prescription and OTC medications and herbal remedies. If you are taking any of these and are depressed or anxious or have any other mood problems, they might be contributing to them. In the case of prescribed drugs, ask your doctor about alternatives. Experiment with discontinuing the use of other products to see if your moods improve.
- If you drink coffee or use other forms of caffeine every day, try going without it to see if you have a withdrawal reaction. If you do, stay off caffeine until you determine how much—if at all—it has been affecting your energy, sleep, and moods. You can then experiment with it to learn how much you can tolerate and what forms most agree with you—maybe you can drink an occasional tea rather than habitual coffee, for example. If you suffer from an anxiety disorder, avoid caffeine in any form. Just go cold turkey and put up with a few days of withdrawal symptoms if you have to.

- Familiarize yourself with the details of the Anti-Inflammatory Diet in Appendix A. Remember: most important is to reduce your consumption of refined, processed, and manufactured food. Go through your refrigerator, freezer, and pantry to identify such products and resolve to phase them out of your life. You have plenty of time in the coming weeks to move your eating habits in the right direction.
- Make a list of friends and acquaintances who have good eating habits. Resolve to spend more time with them.
- Start taking fish oil: 2 to 4 grams a day of a product that provides both EPA and DHA (more of the former). Read labels carefully to make sure you're getting 2 to 4 grams of total omega-3 fatty acids (EPA and DHA), not of oil. Pass up products that include omega-6 or omega-9 fatty acids; you don't need to supplement with them. Buy only brands of fish oil that are "molecularly distilled" or otherwise guaranteed to be free of toxic contaminants. You may have to take three or four capsules twice a day to get the recommended dose. Take them on a full stomach. If you get fish-flavored burps, try keeping the product in the freezer and swallowing frozen capsules.
- Also start taking 2,000 IU of vitamin D daily. You can use either D2 or D3. Note that if your 25-hydroxy-vitamin D level is very low, you might need much higher doses for a few weeks to bring it into the normal range; your physician can advise you on this.
- If you take a daily multivitamin/multimineral supplement, make sure it provides 400 micrograms (mcg) of folic acid, at least 50 milligrams (mg) of vitamin B-6 (pyridoxine), and 50 mcg of vitamin B-12 (cyanocobolamin). If you do not take a daily multivitamin/multimineral supplement, start doing so. To ensure absorption and avoid indigestion, take it after an ample meal.
- If you are not getting some physical activity every day, ask yourself what prevents you from doing so. Try to take a brisk walk every day this week, especially if you are not otherwise exercising.

- Make a list of friends and acquaintances who have good habits of physical activity. Start spending more time with them. Call one up this week and go on a walk together.

Caring for Your Mind

- Start practicing the 4-7-8 breath that I described on pages 146 to 147. Do it at least twice a day, every day from now on, *without fail!* Try it in the morning and at night when you get into bed. You can practice it more often, but for the next four weeks, limit yourself to four breath cycles at a time.

Caring for Your Spirit

- Bring fresh flowers into your home and enjoy their beauty.

Week 3: Planning Long-Term Strategies

This week I'd like you to think about your options for managing anxiety and depression. I also want you to focus on your sleep and dreams. And it's time to take on the challenge of managing negative thoughts.

Caring for Your Body

- If you are taking anti-anxiety medication, tell the physician who prescribed it that you want to get off it. Tell him or her that you are following recommendations to stabilize and improve your moods that include specific anti-anxiety measures. Ask for a written schedule for gradually decreasing the dosage and frequency of the medication; you will not start decreasing it until you are on Week 5 of this program (I'll give you further instructions there). Also commit to checking in with the physician regularly as you wean yourself from the drug(s).

- If you are taking antidepressant medication, think about whether you need it. If you have been on it for more than a year, ask the physician who prescribed it if it is time to try getting off it and using other methods to stabilize and improve your moods. Tell him or her about the program you are following, and if you both agree that it is okay to stop taking medication, ask for a schedule that you can follow for safely decreasing your dosage of the drug *once you have completed all eight weeks.*

- Remember that the strongest evidence we have for nondrug treatments for depression is for dietary supplementation with omega-3 fatty acids and exercise. You've started taking the right dose of fish oil, and I hope your daily physical activity will be greater this week than last. You must maintain regular physical activity not only throughout this program but throughout life.

- Make sure you're getting enough restful sleep. Take a self-test on your sleep hygiene at http://psychologytoday.tests.psychtests.com/take_test.php?idRegTest=1329.
- If you are not getting enough restful sleep, try to identify the reasons. Common ones are too much caffeine, bodily aches and pains, the wrong mattress, noise, stress, worry, and an inability to detach from thoughts that make you anxious. You'll likely need help with the last of these, and in a moment I'll tell you what to do. The others have relatively easy fixes. Make sure your bedroom is completely dark when you are ready to sleep, and get a white-noise generator if you need to mask disturbing sounds. For more ideas, use the search term "sleep" at www.DrWeil.com.
- Try not to use prescription or OTC sleep medications except on rare occasions.
- If you need a sleep aid, experiment with the herbal sedative valerian, 2 capsules or 500 milligrams of a standardized extract twenty minutes before you want to sleep. Or try 2.5 milligrams of melatonin in a sublingual tablet (which dissolves under the tongue). Both are safe for regular use.
- If you cannot improve your sleep with these methods, consider consulting a sleep professional. You can find one through the National Sleep Foundation at www.sleepfoundation.org.
- Experiment with recording your dreams. Keep a notebook by your bed and try to write down everything you remember of them just as you wake. (Or tell them to your bed partner or a recording device.) If negative dreams disturb your sleep or moods, this is another problem to take to a sleep professional.
- Experiment with taking brief daytime naps, ten to twenty minutes in the afternoon, best done lying down in a darkened room. See how napping affects your sleep and emotions.

Caring for Your Mind

- It's time to take on the challenge of managing negative thoughts. If you engage in depressive rumination, first try moving your attention to your breath. Experiment with mantram repetition if that interests you. Read *The Mantram Handbook,* select a phrase you like, and give it a try.
- Also try using a positive mental image as an alternative focus of attention. Read over the section on visualization in chapter 6 and use the resources on visualization in Appendix B if you need help.
- If you cannot get yourself out of repetitive patterns of thought that make you depressed or anxious, consider working with a practitioner of cognitive behavioral therapy. CBT is a time- and cost-efficient method that works.
- Mastery of the 4-7-8 breath is your best protection from anxiety. Keep at it!

Caring for Your Spirit

- Spend some time in nature this week, doing nothing but letting its sights, sounds, and scents fill you. If you can get to a patch of wilderness, great; but you can get as much benefit by walking in a park or garden, watching a sunset, or viewing the night sky. Try to do this most days of the week, especially if you feel blue or stressed.

Week 4: Further Steps

At the end of this week, you will be halfway through the program and will have built the foundation of an emotionally healthy lifestyle. You will continue to advance toward your goal by learning to take better care of your mind and spirit.

Caring for Your Body

- Try to get at least thirty minutes of physical activity at least six days of this week, including a few bursts of activity strenuous enough to get you huffing and puffing.
- Review the natural remedies described in chapter 5 on pages 112 to 121, and pick one that you would like to experiment with. Start using it this week.

Caring for Your Mind

- Read up on positive psychology, using the resources in Appendix B.
- Review these two positive psychology exercises — each of which has been shown to boost happiness — and do the one that is most appealing to you: the *Gratitude Visit,* in which you write an essay of gratitude toward someone who has helped you, then visit that person and read it aloud; or the *Three Good Things* intervention, in which you write down three things that went well, and why, each day for a week.
- How successful have you been with mantram repetition, attending to your breath, or using a mental image to interrupt negative thoughts that make you sad or anxious? If the answer is not very, find a CBT practitioner by going to www.nacbt.org and make an initial appointment.
- Try taking breaks from the news — for instance by not listening to or watching any news programs on radio or television for

two or three days of this week. Note any differences in how you feel.

Caring for Your Spirit

- Make a list of people in your life in whose company you feel more optimistic, more positive, more cheerful, less anxious. Resolve to spend more time with them. Make a date with one of them this week.
- Listen to music that elevates your mood and spirit.

Week 5: Evaluating Progress

Congratulations! You are halfway there. This is a good time to take stock of where you are and where you came from.

- How much have you changed your diet in the past four weeks? Have you reduced your intake of refined, processed, and manufactured food? How many elements of the Anti-Inflammatory Diet have you incorporated into your life? What are you having most trouble giving up? Or adding? Are you more careful about your food selections when you shop and when you eat out?
- Are you regularly taking your daily multivitamin/multimineral supplement, vitamin D, and fish oil?
- Where are you with caffeine? Do you think it has been affecting your moods? Have you tried going without it?
- Are you getting more daily physical activity now than when you started the program? Have you been able to identify and remove obstacles to being more physically active? Found friends to walk with?
- Are you doing the 4-7-8 breath at least twice a day every day? You should be. Are you beginning to notice any effects from it? Does it help you relax or fall asleep?
- What about your sleep? Have you identified anything that keeps you from getting enough good-quality sleep? What corrective action have you taken?
- Have you remembered any dreams?
- Are you inspired to keep flowers in your home more of the time?
- Have you spent more time in nature?
- What has been your experience with managing your thoughts?
- Have you thought about trying CBT? Have you found a therapist? Made an initial appointment?
- Did you find the positive psychology exercise helpful? Will you try another?

- Have you spent time with someone more optimistic and positive than you are?
- Are you using one of the natural remedies I suggested?

I hope you feel you've made progress toward your goal after being on the program for a month. Which assignments have been easiest for you? Which have been hardest? Can you see any changes in your emotional life? Are you ready to move forward?

Caring for Your Body

- If you have been taking anti-anxiety medication and have a schedule to follow for gradually cutting the dose, you can begin to do so this week. If you become anxious as you do this, experiment with valerian or kava (see page 117).
- Be sure to get out in some bright light as many days as you can.
- Treat yourself to a massage this week.

Caring for Your Mind

- It's time to increase to eight breath cycles when you practice the 4-7-8 breath. That will be the most you will ever do in one session. The practice is now eight breath cycles twice a day without fail. You can do the exercise as often as you want. You should be comfortable with it now and can try slowing down your count. I would like you to begin using the 4-7-8 breath whenever you start to feel anxious or stressed.
- How much noise are you exposed to? How does it affect you? What steps can you take to minimize it or protect yourself from it? Check the resources in Appendix B for products that can help.
- How did you respond to taking breaks from the news? Keep experimenting to gain better control of how much of that information you want in your life.

- Pay attention to the choices of media you make. What do you like to read, watch, and listen to for diversion and entertainment? Is the content consistent with the goal(s) you've set for yourself in this program? If not, start to make appropriate changes.

Caring for Your Spirit

- Keep a Gratitude Journal this week. (Maybe you did this as your positive psychology exercise last week; if so, keep it up this week, too.) Dedicate a notebook to this assignment and keep it by your bed. Make mental notes throughout the day of things you have to be grateful for, then enter them briefly in your journal at bedtime. Take a moment to feel grateful.
- Do you have a companion animal? If so, spend more time with it this week and express your gratitude for its presence in your life. If not, give serious thought this week to bringing one into your life.

Week 6: Gaining Momentum

Before you know it, you will have completed this program. You know that you will have to continue the practices I have introduced you to in order to realize their long-term benefits. By now, however, you should have a sense of the many ways that you can influence your emotions and which have most to offer you. Begin to think about how you can stick with them beyond Week 8. And get ready to tackle the problem of information overload.

Caring for Your Body

- If you have ruled out or dealt with any medical problems that might be responsible for suboptimal emotional wellness; if you are phasing out refined, processed, and manufactured food and are following the Anti-Inflammatory Diet as best you can; if you are taking your fish oil and other dietary supplements; if you are getting good physical activity most days of the week; if you are getting enough restful sleep; if you have made any needed changes in your uses of mood-altering drugs; and if you are practicing the 4-7-8 breath as I have instructed, you are doing everything you should be doing on the physical level to attain optimum emotional well-being.
- Keep at it! If you need help with improving your eating habits or exercising regularly, spend more time in the company of people who have the habits you want to develop.
- Try giving and receiving more hugs this week.

Caring for Your Mind

- How do you rate yourself on empathy and compassion? Consider taking an empathy training course. Also consider trying compassion meditation (resources for both are listed in Appendix B).

- It's time to start limiting information overload. Begin by keeping track this week of the amount of time you spend on the phone, on the Internet, on e-mail, texting, etc. (A Google search for "Internet timer" will direct you to software that tracks your time online automatically.) How many times a day do you check e-mail? Pay attention to how often you try to multitask. At the end of this week, look over the record you've kept and think about how easy or difficult it will be for you to limit these activities.

Caring for Your Spirit

- Visit an art museum this week and spend some time with one or more works of art you find beautiful and uplifting.
- Look around your home for objects of beauty and take time to enjoy them. If your living space is deficient in beauty, look for a piece of art or a handicraft that you find pleasing and affordable and bring it into your home. Remember to notice it, enjoy it, and be grateful for its presence.

Week 7: Keeping Your Eyes on the Goal

You're getting close to the finish line. And you have important work to do this week, including setting limits on Internet, e-mail, and mobile-phone use, and choosing a meditation technique to practice.

Caring for Your Body

- If you enjoyed the massage and found it helped your mood, arrange to get one on a regular basis. If it did not meet your expectations, try another form of body work; for example, those who find deep-tissue massage too vigorous may prefer the Trager Approach, with its gentle, rocking motions, or watsu, done in a heated pool.

Caring for Your Mind

- Read over the information on meditation on pages 149 to 151. Look through the resources on meditation in Appendix B and choose one or more to use—a book, an audio program, a website, or a class or group you can join.
- Try your hand at meditation, if only for a few minutes a day. Sit comfortably, relax, do a 4-7-8 breath, then try a method that appeals to you. It can be as simple as following your breath and bringing your attention back to your breath whenever you are aware that it has wandered.
- Try limiting your Internet time this week. Cut the hours you spent on the Internet last week by 25 percent. Use the time you free up for outings in nature, exercise, or activities with friends who make you feel more positive.
- Cut back on the number of times a day you check e-mail. For instance, you might resolve not to do so after a certain hour of the day.

- Also try to cut back on texting and talking on a mobile phone.

Caring for Your Spirit

- Laugh! Who do you know who tends to laugh with you? Invite someone in that category to watch a funny movie with you.
- Locate a laughter group in your area and give it a try this week.

Week 8: The Home Stretch

In the last week of this program, you are going to take a few more important steps toward your goal(s), especially in the realm of caring for your spirit.

Caring for Your Body

- If you have been using one or more of the suggested natural remedies for the past four weeks, you should have some sense of how it is working for you. Can you note any benefits to your moods or well-being? If so, continue using it for another month, then decide whether you want to stay on it, stop it to see if the benefits persist, use it intermittently or only when you feel you need it, or switch to a different remedy.

- If you have been weaning yourself from anti-anxiety medication, you should be well along in that process. If you are having difficulty, be patient. Use the 4-7-8 breath whenever you start to feel anxious.

- If you have been taking prescribed antidepressants and have decided in consultation with your physician that it is a good idea to try getting off them, look over the schedule for decreasing dosage gradually and think about whether you feel confident enough in your progress over the past weeks toward greater emotional stability to start cutting back. You can take as much time with this as you need. You can also stay on the medication if you find that you need it.

Caring for Your Mind

- I have introduced you to methods to manage negative thoughts and get yourself out of cycles of depressive rumination. Please keep practicing those that work best for you, whether mantram repetition, visualization, meditation on the breath, positive psychology exercises, or CBT therapy. The more you work with them, the more effective they become.

- Meditation is a powerful long-term strategy for restructuring the mind and changing brain function. I've given you just a taste of it in this program and don't expect you to have experienced what it can do for you. I urge you to experiment with various forms and styles of meditation until you find one that suits you, and to make it a daily practice.

- I have also given you tips for protecting yourself from the harmful influences of information overload. It takes effort and dedication to put these into practice. Information and communication technology will keep expanding and affecting our lives and minds. Find ways to limit the time you spend with the new devices and media.

- By now the 4-7-8 breath should be part of your daily life and you should begin to notice effects of practicing it. Begin to use it purposefully — for example, to get your mind off cravings, to fall back to sleep if you get up in the middle of the night, or to forestall angry reactions to common annoyances.

- I hope you are being more conscious about mental nutrition and choosing what to read, watch, and listen to with consideration of possible effects on your outlook and mood.

Caring for Your Spirit

- It is now time to practice forgiveness. Are you holding on to anger or resentment toward people who have hurt or wronged you? If so, pick one person for this exercise. Every day this week, try to put yourself in that person's place. Can you understand why they acted as they did? Also consider how the negative feelings you are holding on to stand in the way of your attaining your goal of optimum emotional well-being.

- Before the end of the week, try to let go of those feelings by writing a letter of forgiveness to the person who caused them. You do not have to send the letter—now or ever—unless you are moved to do so. You are doing this for yourself. Put the letter aside. Read it over the next day, making any changes you feel are necessary. Note how you feel as a result of doing this.
- If you realize the emotional value of forgiving, look for other opportunities to practice it.
- Go for a helper's high this week. Lend a hand, do favors. Try some volunteer or service work. (See resources in Appendix B.)
- Expose yourself to silence when you can this week. How does it make you feel? Can you find ways to experience it more frequently?
- How are you doing with social connection? If you need more, look for interest groups you can join, classes to take, activities you enjoy that you can do with others.
- Are you spending more time with people who are emotionally healthy and positive? With people who make you laugh?
- Are you feeling grateful and expressing it? You don't need to keep up with a Gratitude Journal, at least not every day, unless you find it useful. But try to remember to feel grateful for the food on your table when you sit down to meals, for your health, for all that supports you and contributes to your well-being. And maybe thank a special friend for being in your life. Remember that training yourself to feel and express gratitude will move your set point for happiness in the right direction.

A Final Assignment

- Go back to the questions I asked in Week 1 about your emotional health, lifestyle, and personal traits. Answer them again. Note how your answers have changed as the result of completing this program.

Week 9 and Beyond

During this week — and all the weeks to come — use the lessons you have learned about yourself over the course of the 8-week program to refine and enhance your lifestyle.

Keep in mind that we are most similar to one another when it comes to our physical needs. The "body" recommendations in the program are, I believe, suitable for nearly everyone. Following an anti-inflammatory diet made up of unprocessed foods, taking regular moderate exercise, practicing stress reduction, and using prudent supplementation make sense for all of us.

Yet even here, there is plenty of room for sensible experimentation. A friend of mine in his midsixties, struggling with low mood, understood that exercise was crucial to emotional well-being but had simply been unable to maintain interest in any particular workout regimen. By chance one day a relative asked him to hit a few balls on a tennis court, something he had never done in his life. Tennis became his path to a new self, contributing to his well-being in ways that jogging, aerobics, and weightlifting never had. In addition to satisfying his need for exercise, tennis gave him sunlight and fresh air, friendship, travel opportunities, and even a measure of recognition — he became a champion player in his senior circuit, gaining a sense of accomplishment he had missed since retiring from a competitive business. In short, it lifted his mood dramatically, and it all happened because he was willing, one afternoon, to try something new.

In the areas of mind and spirit, the glorious diversity of individual needs is much greater, and it is worth noting Ralph Waldo Emerson's words: "All life is an experiment. The more experiments you make the better." In exploring the range of mental and spiritual endeavors that can lead human beings to happiness and fulfillment, some of you will find it best to work within established psychological and spiritual disciplines that tell you what to do and not do. Others will prefer looser organizing principles that encourage you to make your own rules and be comfortable with uncertainty.

Whatever your personal style, I firmly believe that the program I have outlined here covers the basics—the necessary aspects of human physical, mental, and spiritual sustenance that, if attended to, can improve your mood and emotional well-being dramatically. Once you reach a new, better equilibrium, it will be up to you to find the particulars of how best to maintain, express, and improve it.

Take heart, stay on the path, experiment to discover what works best for you, and lend a hand to others you may encounter on the way. I wish you all success in the journey.

Acknowledgments

B rad Lemley, editorial director of Weil Lifestyle, LLC, alerted me to the fact that depression is the subject of a great majority of questions addressed to me at www.DrWeil.com. When I mentioned this to my agent, Richard Pine, he encouraged me to write a book on the topic and helped me find a home for it at Little, Brown and Company. I am indebted to my editor there, Tracy Behar, to the whole Little, Brown team, to Richard Pine, and to Brad Lemley. I have become significantly happier as a result of writing this book and am grateful to everyone who inspired and supported the project.

Brad is also a professional science writer with a long-standing interest in brain research and psychology. He provided invaluable assistance in finding information I needed and supplying me with material that I have used. It has been a pleasure to work with him.

Susan Bulzoni Levenberg, Brad's colleague at Weil Lifestyle who manages my social media, requested first-person accounts of experiences with the treatments and strategies that I recommend. She sorted through the many responses, selecting ones most relevant. I thank her for that assistance and, of course, am very grateful to all those persons who allowed me to tell their stories in this book.

A number of friends and colleagues gave me ideas and suggestions:

Dr. Victoria Maizes, Dr. Bernard Beitman, Dr. Jim Nicolai, Dr. Russell Greenfield, Dr. Ulka Agarwal, Dr. Rubin Naiman, Dr. Tieraona Low Dog, Winifred Rosen, Charris Ford, Betty Anne Sarver, and Richard Pine. Dr. Brian Becker devoted a great deal of his time to helping me compile the reference notes. He also proofread the manuscript, and I thank him for all of his effort.

Special thanks are due to my business partner, Richard Baxter, who managed my schedule to carve out writing time and helped plan promotion of the book, and to my dedicated executive assistant, Nancy Olmstead. I also acknowledge the constant devotion of Ajax and Asha, my canine companions, who stayed by my side as I wrote.

Appendix A

The Anti-Inflammatory Diet

It is becoming increasingly clear that chronic inflammation is the root cause of many serious illnesses—including heart disease, many cancers, and Alzheimer's disease. We all know inflammation on the surface of the body as local redness, heat, swelling, and pain. It is the cornerstone of the body's healing response, bringing more nourishment and immune activity to a site of injury or infection. But when inflammation persists or serves no purpose, it damages the body and causes illness. Stress, lack of exercise, genetic predisposition, and exposure to toxins (like secondhand tobacco smoke) can all contribute to chronic inflammation, and dietary choices play a big role as well. Learning how specific foods influence the inflammatory process is the best strategy for containing it and reducing long-term disease risks.

The Anti-Inflammatory Diet is not a diet in the popular sense—it is not intended as a weight-loss program (although people can and do lose weight on it), nor is it an eating plan to stay on for a limited period of time. Rather, it is a way of selecting and preparing foods based on scientific knowledge of how they can help your body maintain optimum health. Along with influencing inflammation, this diet will provide steady energy and ample vitamins, minerals, essential fatty acids, dietary fiber, and protective phytonutrients.

You can also adapt your existing recipes according to these anti-inflammatory diet principles:

General Diet Tips

- Aim for variety.
- Include as much fresh food as possible.
- Minimize your consumption of processed foods and fast food.
- Eat an abundance of fruits and vegetables.
- Limit sweets of all kinds.

Caloric Intake

- Most adults need to consume between 2,000 and 3,000 calories a day.
- Women and smaller and less active people need fewer calories.
- Men and bigger and more active people need more calories.
- If you are eating the appropriate number of calories for your level of activity, your weight should not fluctuate greatly.
- The distribution of calories you take in should be as follows: 40 to 50 percent from carbohydrates, 30 percent from fat, and 20 to 30 percent from protein.
- Try to include carbohydrates, fat, and protein at each meal.

Carbohydrates

- On a 2,000-calorie-a-day diet, women should consume between 160 and 200 grams of carbohydrates a day.
- Men should consume between 240 and 300 grams of carbohydrates a day.
- The majority of carbohydrates consumed should be in the form of less-refined, less-processed foods with a low glycemic load.

- Reduce your consumption of foods made with flour and sugar, especially breads and most packaged snack foods (including chips and pretzels).
- Eat more whole grains, such as brown rice and bulgur wheat, in which the grain is intact or in a few large pieces. These are preferable to whole-wheat-flour products, which have roughly the same glycemic index as white-flour products.
- Eat more beans, winter squashes, and sweet potatoes.
- Cook pasta al dente and eat it in moderation.
- Avoid products made with high-fructose corn syrup.

Fat

- On a 2,000-calorie-a-day diet, 600 calories can come from fat—that is, about 67 grams. This should be in a ratio of 1:2:1 of saturated to monounsaturated to polyunsaturated fat.
- Reduce your intake of saturated fat by eating less butter, cream, high-fat cheese, unskinned chicken and fatty meats, and products made with palm kernel oil.
- Use extra-virgin olive oil as your main cooking oil. If you want a neutral-tasting oil, use expeller-pressed, organic canola oil. Organic, high-oleic, expeller-pressed versions of sunflower and safflower oils are also acceptable.
- Avoid regular safflower and sunflower oils, corn oil, cottonseed oil, and mixed vegetable oils.
- Strictly avoid margarine, vegetable shortening, and all products listing them as ingredients. Strictly avoid all products made with partially hydrogenated oils of any kind.
- Include in your diet avocados and nuts, especially walnuts, cashews, almonds, and nut butters made from these nuts.
- For omega-3 fatty acids, eat salmon (preferably fresh or frozen wild or canned sockeye), sardines packed in water or olive oil, herring, and black cod (sablefish, butterfish); omega-3 fortified eggs; and hemp seeds and flaxseeds (preferably freshly ground).

Protein
- On a 2,000-calorie-a-day diet, your daily intake of protein should be between 80 and 120 grams. Eat less protein if you have liver or kidney problems, allergies, or autoimmune disease.
- Decrease your consumption of animal protein except for fish and high-quality natural cheese and yogurt.
- Eat more vegetable protein, especially from beans in general and soybeans in particular. Become familiar with the range of whole soy foods available and find ones you like.

Fiber
- Try to eat 40 grams of fiber a day. You can achieve this by increasing your consumption of fruits (especially berries), vegetables (especially beans), and whole grains.
- Ready-made cereals can be good fiber sources, but read labels to make sure they give you at least 4 and preferably 5 grams of fiber per one-ounce serving.

Phytonutrients
- To get maximum natural protection against age-related diseases (including cardiovascular disease, cancer, and neurodegenerative disease) as well as against environmental toxicity, eat a variety of fruits, vegetables, and mushrooms.
- Choose fruits and vegetables from all parts of the color spectrum, especially berries, tomatoes, orange and yellow fruits, and dark leafy greens.
- Choose organic produce whenever possible. Learn which conventionally grown crops are most likely to carry pesticide residues and avoid them. (Go to http://www.ewg.org, the website of the Environmental Working Group, for their lists of the Dirty Dozen and Clean Fifteen—the most and least contaminated crops.)
- Eat cruciferous (cabbage-family) vegetables regularly.
- Include whole soy foods in your diet.

- Drink tea instead of coffee, especially good-quality white, green, or oolong tea.
- If you drink alcohol, use red wine preferentially.
- Enjoy plain dark chocolate in moderation (look for a minimum cocoa content of 70 percent).

Vitamins and Minerals

The best way to obtain all of your daily vitamins, minerals, and micronutrients is by eating a diet high in fresh foods with an abundance of fruits and vegetables.

In addition, supplement your diet with the following antioxidant cocktail:

- Vitamin C, 200 milligrams a day.
- Vitamin E, 400 IU of natural mixed tocopherols (d-alpha-tocopherol with other tocopherols or, better, a minimum of 80 milligrams of natural mixed tocopherols and tocotrienols).
- Selenium, 200 micrograms of an organic (yeast-bound) form.
- Mixed carotenoids, 10,000–15,000 IU daily.
- Antioxidants can be most conveniently taken as part of a daily multivitamin/multimineral supplement that also provides at least 400 micrograms of folic acid and 2,000 IU of vitamin D. It should contain no iron (unless you are female and having regular menstrual periods) and no preformed vitamin A (retinol). Take these supplements with your largest meal.

Other Dietary Supplements

- If you are not eating oily fish at least twice a week, take supplemental fish oil in capsule or liquid form (2–3 grams a day of a product containing both EPA and DHA). Look for molecularly distilled products certified to be free of heavy metals and other contaminants.

- Talk to your doctor about going on low-dose aspirin therapy, two baby aspirins a day (162 milligrams).
- If you are not regularly eating ginger and turmeric, consider taking these in supplemental form.
- Add CoQ10 to your daily regimen: 60–100 milligrams of a softgel form taken with your largest meal.
- If you are prone to metabolic syndrome, take alpha-lipoic acid, 200–400 milligrams a day.

Water

- Drink pure water or drinks that are mostly water (tea, very diluted fruit juice, sparkling water with lemon) throughout the day.
- Use bottled water or get a home water purifier if your tap water tastes of chlorine or other contaminants, or if you live in an area where the water is known or suspected to be contaminated.

Appendix B

SUGGESTED READING, RESOURCES, AND SUPPLIES

Books

Baumel, Syd. *Dealing with Depression Naturally: Complementary and Alternative Therapies for Restoring Emotional Health*. New York: McGraw Hill, 2000.

Challem, Jack. *The Food-Mood Solution: All-Natural Ways to Banish Anxiety, Depression, Anger, Stress, Overeating, and Alcohol and Drug Problems—and Feel Good Again*. Hoboken, N.J.: John Wiley & Sons, 2007.

Easwaran, Eknath. *The Mantram Handbook: A Practical Guide to Choosing Your Mantram and Calming Your Mind*. Tomales, Calif.: Nilgiri Press, 2008.

Haidt, Jonathan. *The Happiness Hypothesis: Finding Modern Truth in Ancient Wisdom*. New York: Basic Books, 2006.

Horwitz, Allan V., and Jerome C. Wakefield. *The Loss of Sadness: How Psychiatry Transformed Normal Sorrow into Depressive Disorder*. Oxford: Oxford University Press, 2007.

Ilardi, Stephen S., PhD. *The Depression Cure: The 6-Step Program to Beat Depression Without Drugs*. Cambridge: Da Capo Press, 2009.

Larson, Joan Mathews, PhD. *Depression-Free, Naturally: 7 Weeks to Eliminating Anxiety, Despair, Fatigue, and Anger from Your Life*. New York: Ballantine Books, 1999.

Nhat Hanh, Thich. *Happiness: Essential Mindfulness Practices*. Berkeley, Calif.: Parallax Press, 2009.

Prochnik, George. *In Pursuit of Silence: Listening for Meaning in a World of Noise*. New York: Doubleday, 2010.

Rossman, Martin, MD. *The Worry Solution: Using Breakthrough Brain Science to Turn Stress and Anxiety into Confidence and Happiness*. New York: Crown Archetype, 2010.

Schachter, Michael B., MD, and Deborah Mitchell. *What Your Doctor May Not Tell You About Depression: The Breakthrough Integrative Approach for Effective Treatment*. New York: Wellness Central, 2006.

Seligman, Martin E. P. *Learned Optimism*. New York: Alfred A. Knopf, 1991.

Solomon, Andrew. *The Noonday Demon: An Atlas of Depression*. New York: Scribner, 2001.

Sood, Amit, MD, MSc. *Train Your Brain, Engage Your Heart, Transform Your Life: A Two Step Program to Enhance Attention; Decrease Stress; Cultivate Peace, Joy, and Resilience; and Practice Presence with Love*. Rochester, Minn.: Morning Dew Publications, LLC, 2010.

Watters, Ethan. *Crazy Like Us: The Globalization of the American Psyche*. New York: Free Press, 2010.

Weil, Andrew. *8 Weeks to Optimum Health: A Proven Program for Taking Full Advantage of Your Body's Natural Healing Power*, rev. ed. New York: Ballantine Books, 2006.

Weil, Andrew. *Natural Health, Natural Medicine: The Complete Guide to Wellness and Self-Care for Optimum Health*, rev. ed. Boston: Houghton Mifflin, 2004.

Weil, Andrew. *Spontaneous Healing: How to Discover and Enhance Your Body's Natural Ability to Maintain and Heal Itself.* New York: Ballantine Books, 2000.

Weil, Andrew, and Rosie Daley. *The Healthy Kitchen: Recipes for a Better Body, Life, and Spirit.* New York: Knopf, 2002.

Websites

My website, www.drweil.com, has a great deal of content on depression, as well as content related to therapies recommended in this book, including dietary supplements, exercise, meditation, breathing techniques, and more. Use the search function to find specific articles and videos. Click "Free Health Emails from Dr. Weil" on the homepage to subscribe to *Dr. Weil's Body, Mind and Spirit Newsletter,* which offers weekly email tips and inspiration.

I also have a dedicated *Spontaneous Happiness* website that provides a comprehensive step-by-step program to improve emotional health. Visit www.SpontaneousHappiness.com for more information.

The website of the Arizona Center for Integrative Medicine, www .AzCIM.org, has information about integrative medicine and a physician locator on the homepage.

Other websites with depression content that meets my criteria for quality include:

Medicinenet
www.medicinenet.com

National Institute of Mental Health
www.nimh.nih.gov

Netdoctor.co.uk
www.netdoctor.co.uk

WebMD.com
www.webmd.com

Recommended websites with content related to specific therapies recommended in this book include:

Cognitive-Behavioral Therapy:

National Association of Cognitive-Behavioral Therapists
www.nacbt.org

Compassion Training:

Providers and Classes
www.training-classes.com/learn/_k/c/o/m/compassion/

Empathy Training:

The Empathy Training Console
http://empathytrainingconsole.com/

Forgiveness:

Stanford Forgiveness Project
http://learningtoforgive.com

Gratitude:

Spirituality and Practice
www.spiritualityandpractice.com/practices/practices.php?id=11

Laughter Clubs:

Laughter Yoga International
www.laughteryoga.org

Meditation:

Insight Meditation Center (Vipassana)
www.insightmeditationcenter.org

Project Meditation
www.project-meditation.org

Susan Piver (meditation resources)
www.susanpiver.com

Mindfulness Training and MBSR:

Mindful Living Programs
www.mindfullivingprograms.com

Physical Activity:

Mayo Clinic (fitness section)
www.mayoclinic.com/health/fitness/MY00396

Positive Psychology:

Positive Psychology Center
www.ppc.sas.upenn.edu

Visualization:

Academy for Guided Imagery
www.acadgi.com

Visualization Exercises
www.key-hypnosis.com

Audio Programs

Jon Kabat-Zinn, "Mindfulness for Beginners," Sounds True audio edition, 2007.

Andrew Weil, "Breathing: The Master Key to Self Healing," Sounds True audio edition, 1999.

Andrew Weil and Jon Kabat-Zinn, "Meditation for Optimum Health: How to Use Mindfulness and Breathing to Heal Your Body and Refresh Your Mind," Sounds True audio edition, 2001.

Andrew Weil and Rubin Naiman, "Healthy Sleep: Wake Up Refreshed and Energized with Proven Practices for Optimum Sleep," Sounds True audio edition, 2007.

The first Integrative Mental Health Conference was held in Phoenix, Arizona, on March 22–24, 2010, and featured presentations by the leaders in the field. CDs and DVDs are available from www.conferencerecording .com. Type "integrative mental health" into the search box.

I also recommend CDs and audio downloads from psychotherapist Belleruth Naparstek, especially those titled "Depression," "Relieve Stress," and "Healthful Sleep." These and other resources are available at her website, www.healthjourneys.com.

Dietary Supplements

I recommend and use Weil Nutritional Supplements brand vitamins, minerals, and supplements, which are available from DrWeil.com. I have developed these science-based formulations and oversee their production. Go to www.drweil.com and click on the "Marketplace" tab or the "Vitamin Advisor" link. These products are also available at many specialty health stores.

Products that align with recommendations in this book include:

Antioxidant & Multivitamin
Mood Support
Omega-3 Support

(All of my after-tax profits from royalties from sales of these products go to the Weil Foundation, www.WeilFoundation.org, a nonprofit organization that supports the advance of integrative medicine through education, research, and public policy reform.)

Other products that also meet my specifications for quality:

Standardized extracts of ashwagandha, *Rhodiola rosea,* St. John's wort, and valerian:
Nature's Way Products, Inc.
3051 West Maple Loop Dr., Suite 125
Lehi, UT 84043
www.naturesway.com

Fish oil capsules and liquids:
Nordic Naturals, Inc.
94 Hangar Way
Watsonville, CA 95076
www.nordicnaturals.com

Extracts of holy basil, rhodiola, and turmeric:
New Chapter, Inc.
22 High St.
Brattleboro, VT 05301
www.newchapter.com

Melatonin sublingual tablets:
Source Naturals
23 Janis Way
Scotts Valley, CA 95066
www.sourcenaturals.com

SAMe:
Nature Made
P.O. Box 9606
Mission Hills, CA 91346
www.naturemade.com/products/segments/SAMe

Other Products
Light box (free of wavelengths that may cause retinal damage):
Lo-LIGHT Desk Lamp, model D 120
Sunnex Biotechnologies
Suite 657-167 Lombard Ave.
Winnipeg, MB Canada R3B-0V3
1-877-778-6639
www.sunnexbiotech.com

Noise-cancellation headphones:
Bose QuietComfort 15 Acoustic Noise Cancelling Headphones
Bose Corporation
The Mountain
Framingham, MA 01701
1-800-999-2673
www.bose.com

White-noise generator:
Marpac SleepMate 980A Electro-Mechanical Sound Conditioner
Marpac Corporation
P.O. Box 560
Rocky Point, NC 28457
1-800-999-6962
www.marpac.com

Notes

Introduction

4: **The Harvard psychologist Daniel Gilbert has spent more than a decade studying just how abysmal human beings are at predicting which future events will make them happy:** "The Science of Happiness: A Talk with Daniel Gilbert," introduction by John Brockman, www.edge.org/3rd_culture/gilbert06 /gilbert06_index.html.

7: **Cardiologists now know that loss of heart-rate variability is an early sign of disease:** E. Kristal et al., "Heart Rate Variability in Health and Disease," *Scand J Environ Health* 2 (April 21, 1995): 85–95. See also editorial by J. M. Karemaker and K. I. Lie, "Heart Rate Variability: A Telltale of Health or Disease," *European Heart J* 21 (March 2000): 435–37, www.heartmath .org.

8: **Ramakrishna Paramahansa (1836–1886), a famous Indian saint:** Walther G. Neevel Jr., "The Transformation of Sri Ramakrishna," in *Hinduism: New Essays in the History of Religions,* edited by Bardwell L. Smith (The Netherlands: E. J. Brill, 1976), 53–97. See also Peter Holleran, "Ramakrishna Paramahansa—

God-Intoxicated Saint," www.mountainrunnerdoc.com/articles /article/2291157/31005.htm.

CHAPTER 1. What Is Emotional Well-Being?

22: **Yet enforced, almost bullying cheerfulness dominates our culture:** Barbara Ehrenreich, *Bright-Sided: How the Relentless Promotion of Positive Thinking Has Undermined America* (New York: Metropolitan Books, 2009).

22: **"The president almost demanded optimism," noted Bush's secretary of state Condoleezza Rice:** Ehrenreich, *Bright-Sided,* 10. See also Richard Pine, "Bush's Toxic Optimism," *Huffington Post,* September 16, 2007, www.huffingtonpost.com /richard-pine/bushs-toxic-optimism_b_64616.html.

22: **One [study], from 2004, notes:** Yukiko Uchida et al., "Cultural Constructions of Happiness: Theory and Empirical Evidence," *J Happiness Studies* 5 (2004): 223–39.

22: **Other scholarly articles report significant differences from country to country in rates of reported happiness:** Roya Rohani Rad, "Happiness: A Literature Review of Cross Cultural Implications," November 2010, www.selfknowledgebase.com/files /happinessliteraturereview.pdf.

CHAPTER 2. An Epidemic of Depression

25: **The World Health Organization predicts that by 2030 more people worldwide will be affected by depression than by any other health condition:** "Depression Looms as Global Crisis," BBC News, September 2, 2009, http://news.bbc.co.uk/2/hi /health/8230549.stm.

25: **The number of Americans taking antidepressant drugs doubled in the decade from 1996 to 2005:** Amanda Gardner, "Antidepressant Use in U.S. Has Almost Doubled," *Healthday,* August 3, 2009, http://health.usnews.com/health-news/family

-health/brain-and-behavior/articles/2009/08/03/antidepressant
-use-in-us-has-almost-doubled.

25: **Today an astonishing one in ten people in the United States,
including millions of children, is on one or more of these medications:** Katharine Kam, "Can Antidepressants Work for Me?"
WebMD, February 20, 2011, www.webmd.com/depression
/features/are-antidepressants-effective.

26: **the *Diagnostic and Statistical Manual of Mental Disorders* (DSM):** *Diagnostic and Statistical Manual of Mental Disorders, Fourth Edition, Text Revision* (DSM-IV-TR), published by the
American Psychiatric Association, 2000. DSM-V will appear in
2012.

26: **The current edition of the DSM gives specific criteria for the
diagnosis of this most severe form of depression:** DSM-IV-TR.

27: **The novelist William Styron, author of *Sophie's Choice,* provides:** William Styron, *Darkness Visible: A Memoir of Madness*
(New York: Vintage, 1992), 50.

28: **The English writer Aldous Huxley wrote of it:** Aldous Huxley,
Beyond the Mexique Bay: A Traveler's Guide (New York: Harper
and Brothers, 1934).

29: **According to the DSM's classification, I would have been
diagnosed with dysthymic disorder, the commonest form of
mild to moderate depression:** DSM-IV-TR.

30: **A prominent health website notes that in one group surveyed:** "The Relationship Between Depression and Anxiety,"
HealthyPlace.com, January 13, 2009, www.healthyplace.com
/depression/main/relationship-between-depression-and-anxiety
/menu-id-68/.

30: **Women are twice as likely as men to experience depression:**
Stephanie A. Riolo et al., "Findings from the National Health
and Nutrition Examination Survey III," *Am J Pub Health* 65,
no. 6 (June 2005): 998–1000.

31: **We know also that depression commonly coexists with physical illness:** National Institute of Mental Health, 2002, www.nimh.nih.gov/health/publications/depression/complete-index.shtml.

31: **Nevertheless, experts on aging agree that depression is not a normal consequence of growing older:** National Institute of Mental Health.

31: **The National Institute of Mental Health reports that in any given year, 4 percent of adolescents in our society suffer severe depression:** National Institute of Mental Health.

31: **Depression is also being diagnosed much more frequently in preteens than ever before:** Harvard University study reported in *Harvard Mental Health Newsletter,* February 2002, www.health.harvard.edu/newsweek/Depression_in_Children_Part_I.htm. See also: www.about-teen-depression.com/teen-depression.html; "Depression Facts and Stats," www.upliftprogram.com/depression_stats.html#4; "Depression in Children and Adolescents Fact Sheet," National Alliance on Mental Illness, July 2010, www.nami.org/Template.cfm?Section=by_illness&template=/ContentManagement/ContentDisplay.cfm&ContentID=17623; E. R. Cox et al., "Trends in the Prevalence of Chronic Medication Use in Children: 2002–2005," *Pediatrics* 122, no. 5 (November 2008): e1053–61, pediatrics.aappublications.org/cgi/content/abstract/122/5/e1053.

31: **Along with attention deficit hyperactivity disorder (ADHD) and the autistic disorders, depression accounts for the unprecedented, widespread use of prescribed psychiatric drugs by our young people:** Harvard University study reported in *Harvard Mental Health Newsletter,* February 2002, www.health.harvard.edu/newsweek/Depression_in_Children_Part_I.htm. See also: www.about-teen-depression.com/teen-depression.html; "Depression Facts and Stats," www.upliftprogram.com/depression_stats.html#4; and Cox et al., "Trends," e1053–61.

32: **In 1996, the pharmaceutical industry spent $32 million on DTC antidepressant ads; by 2005, that had nearly quadrupled, to $122 million:** Liz Szabo, "Number of Americans Taking Antidepressants Doubles," *USA Today*, August 4, 2009, www.usatoday.com/news/health/2009-08-03-antidepressants_N.htm.

32: **More than 164 million antidepressant prescriptions were written in 2008, totaling $9.6 billion in US sales:** "Study: Antidepressant Lift May Be All in Your Head," USAToday.com, January 5, 2010, www.usatoday.com/news/health/2010-01-06-antidepressants06_ST_N.htm.

33: ***Crazy Like Us:*** Ethan Watters, *Crazy Like Us: The Globalization of the American Psyche* (New York: Free Press, 2010).

33: **A Nigerian man…"something akin to loneliness":** Watters, *Crazy*, 195.

33: **Over the past decade, however, a massive marketing campaign launched in Japan:** Watters, *Crazy*, 225.

34: **The fact that DTC advertising is illegal in Japan was little impediment:** Watters, *Crazy*, 187–248.

35: **A study published in the April 2007 issue of the *Archives of General Psychiatry:*** Jerome C. Wakefield et al., "Extending the Bereavement Exclusion for Major Depression to Other Losses: Evidence from the National Comorbidity Survey," *Arch Gen Psychiat* 64, no. 4 (April 2007): 433–40.

35: **the rate [of depression] has more than doubled....It is also going up in the rest of the developed world:** W. M. Compton et al., "Changes in the Prevalence of Major Depression and Comorbid Substance Use Disorders in the United States Between 1991–1992 and 2001–2002," *Am J Psychiat* 163, no. 12 (December 2006): 2141–47.

37: **the same study reports that the day-to-day sense of how happy one feels ("positive feelings") is almost entirely unconnected to income level:** Ed Diener et al., "Wealth and Happiness Across the World: Material Prosperity Predicts Life Evaluation, Whereas

Psychosocial Prosperity Predicts Positive Feeling," *J Pers Soc Psychol* 99, no. 1 (2010): 52–61.

37: **The risk of developing major depression has increased tenfold since World War II:** Martin E. P. Seligman and In J. Buie, "'Me' Decades Generate Depression: Individualism Erodes Commitment to Others," *APA Monitor* 19, no. 18 (October 1988): 18.

37: **People who live in poorer countries have a lower risk of depression than those in industrialized nations:** "Unipolar Depressive Disorders World Map," http://en.wikipedia.org/wiki/File:Unipolar_depressive_disorders_world_map_-_DALY_-_WHO2004.svg.

37: **In modernized countries, depression rates are higher for city dwellers than for rural residents:** JiamLi Wang, "Rural–Urban Differences in the Prevalence of Major Depression and Associated Impairment," *Soc Psychiat and Psychiat Epidemiol* 39, no. 1 (2004): 19–25.

37: **In general, countries with lifestyles that are farthest removed from modern standards have the lowest rates of depression:** "Unipolar Depressive Disorders World Map."

37: **Within the United States, the rate of depression among members of the Old Order Amish:** J. A. Egeland and A. M. Hostetter, "Amish Study, I: Affective Disorders Among the Amish, 1976–1980," *Am J Psychiat* 140, no. 1 (January 1983): 56–61.

37: **Hunter-gatherer societies in the modern world have extremely low rates of depression:** Chantal D. Young, "Therapeutic Lifestyle Change: A Brief Psychoeducational Intervention for the Prevention of Depression," submitted to the graduate degree program in Psychology and the Graduate Faculty of the University of Kansas in partial fulfillment of the requirements for the degree of Doctor of Philosophy, August 27, 2009, 31, http://kuscholarworks.ku.edu/dspace/bitstream/1808/5946/1/Young_ku_0099D_10545_DATA_1.pdf.

38: **"neither of these pre-modern cultures has depression at any-thing like the prevalence we do":** Martin E. P. Seligman and R. E. Ingram, eds., "Why Is There So Much Depression Today? The Waxing of the Individual and the Waning of the Commons," *Contemporary Psychological Approaches to Depression: Theory, Research, and Treatment* (New York: Plenum Publishing, 1989–1990), 1–9.

38: **"The more 'modern' a society's way of life, the higher its rate of depression. . . . The human body was never designed for the modern post-industrial environment":** Stephen Ilardi, *The Depression Cure* (Cambridge, Mass.: Da Capo Press, 2009), 6.

39: **Agriculture began ten thousand years ago, and as recently as 1801, 95 percent of Americans still lived on farms:** www .landinstitute.org/vnews/display.v/ART/2004/04/08 /4076b2169776a.

39: **And before the advent of industrial agriculture, farmers lived far healthier lives than most of us today:** Ilardi, *Depression Cure,* 122.

39: **The term *nature deficit disorder* has recently entered the popular vocabulary:** Richard Louv, *Lost Child in the Woods: Saving Our Children from Nature-Deficit Disorder* (Chapel Hill, N.C.: Algonquin Books, 2005).

40: **Hunter-gatherers and other "primitive" peoples do not develop the deficits of vision:** www.physorg.com/news 168157251.html.

42: **More than twenty studies support a link between depression and creativity:** www.cnn.com/2008/HEALTH/conditions/10 /07/creativity.depression/index.html.

42: **Clinical psychologists see rumination as a "way of respond-ing to distress that involves repetitively focusing on the symptoms of distress, and on its possible causes and conse-quences":** S. Nolen-Hoeksema et al., "Rethinking Rumination," *Persp Psychol Sci* 3 (2000): 400–424.

43: **a 2010 *New York Times Magazine* article titled "Depression's Upside":** Jonah Lehrer, *New York Times Magazine*, February 28, 2010, 41, www.nytimes.com/2010/02/28/magazine/28depression-t .html.

44: **"Do you not see how necessary a World of Pains and troubles is to school an Intelligence and make it a soul?":** *John Keats, Selected Letters*, Robert Gittings, ed. (New York: Oxford University Press USA, 2009), xiii.

CHAPTER 3. The Need for a New Approach to Mental Health

45: **In 1977, the journal *Science* published a provocative article:** George L. Engel, "The Need for a New Medical Model: A Challenge for Biomedicine," *Science* 196, no. 4286 (April 8, 1977): 129–35.

48: **In 1980, the American Psychiatric Association radically revised the *Diagnostic and Statistical Manual-III* (DSM-III) to be in accord with the biomedical model:** www.allacademic .com/meta/p_mla_apa_research_citation/1/7/5/4/0/p175408 _index.html.

49: **In 1921, Otto Loewi (1873–1961), a German pharmacologist, demonstrated that nerve cells (neurons) communicate by releasing chemicals:** Renato M. E. Sabbatini, "Neurons and Synapses: The History of Their Discovery," chapter 5, "Chemical Transmission," *Brain & Mind* 17 (2003), www.cerebromente.org .br/n17/history/neurons5_i.htm.

51: **The first antidepressant drug was discovered serendipitously in 1952:** Joseph A. Lieberman, "History of the Use of Antidepressants in Primary Care," "Primary Care Companion," *J Clin Psychiat* 5, S.7 (2003): 6–10.

52: **Amazon sells nearly three thousand books with the word [serotonin] in the title:** Keyword search in August 2010 by author for *serotonin* in Books section of Amazon.com.

53: In fact, a new pharmaceutical known as tianeptine—sold in France and other European countries under the trade name Coaxil—has been shown to be as effective as Prozac: Sharon Begley, "The Depressing News About Antidepressants," *Newsweek Online* (January 29, 2010), www.newsweek.com/2010/01/28 /the-depressing-news-about-antidepressants.html.

53: As psychology professor Irving Kirsch of the University of Hull in England told *Newsweek:* Begley, "Depressing News."

53: The first such analysis, published in 1998: Begley, "Depressing News."

54: In April 2002, the *Journal of the American Medical Association (JAMA)* published the results of a large randomized controlled study: Wayne Jonas et al., "St. John's Wort and Depression," *JAMA* 288, no. 4 (April 2002): 446–49. See also: http://nccam.nih.gov/news/2002/stjohnswort/q-and-a.htm.

54: Zoloft also worked no better than the placebo: Begley, "Depressing News."

54: Irving Kirsch summarized the growing body of evidence against SSRIs in his 2010 book: *The Emperor's New Drugs: Exploding the Antidepressant Myth* (New York: Basic Books, 2010).

54: the most recent analysis, published in the January 6, 2010, issue of *JAMA:* Jay C. Fournier et al., "Antidepressant Drug Effects and Depression Severity: A Patient-Level Meta-analysis," *JAMA* 303, no. 1 (January 5, 2010): 47–53.

54: About 13 percent of people with depression have very severe symptoms: Begley, "Depressing News."

54: One of the authors of the *JAMA* paper, Steven D. Hollon, PhD, of Vanderbilt University, has said: Begley, "Depressing News."

55: Loneliness, for example, is a powerful predictor of depression: R. A. Schoevers et al., "Risk Factors for Depression in Later Life: Results of a Prospective Community Based Study (AMSTEL)," *J Affect Disord* 59, no. 2 (August 2000): 127–37.

57: **I quoted Albert Einstein on the subject of conceptual models:** The quote is from Einstein and Infeld, *Evolution of Physics* (Cambridge, UK: Cambridge University Press, 1938), 152.

59: **individuals trained in meditation have different brain activity from those without such training:** Britta K. Hölzel et al., "Mindfulness Practice Leads to Increases in Regional Brain Matter Density," *Psychiat Res Neuroimaging* 191, no. 1 (January 30, 2011): 36–43.

CHAPTER 4. Integrating Eastern and Western Psychology

61: **Lewis Mehl-Madrona:** *Coyote Medicine* (New York: Simon and Schuster, 1997).

62: **"The Lakota language does not have a concept of strictly mental health":** Lewis Mehl-Madrona, personal communication and lecture content, March 2010.

62: **"In these ways of thinking of the mind and mental health, the *community* is the basic unit of study, not the individual":** Mehl-Madrona communication.

64: **Mind and Life XV, held in 2007 at Emory University in Atlanta:** "Mind and Life XV," www.mindandlife.org/dialogues /past-conferences/ml15/.

64: **"mindfulness-based therapies, along with techniques to enhance compassion, may prove especially useful in the treatment of depression":** "Mind and Life XV," www.mindandlife .org/dialogues/past-conferences/ml15/.

65: **Davidson's studies, along with those of others, demonstrate that neuroplasticity is a fundamental characteristic of our brains:** Richard Davidson and Antoine Lutz, "Buddha's Brain: Neuroplasticity and Meditation," *IEEE Signal Processing Magazine* 25, no. 1 (January, 2008): 174–76.

66: **In a January 2007 interview, Ricard told the British newspaper *The Independent*:** www.independent.co.uk/news/uk/this -britain/the-happiest-man-in-the-world-433063.html.

66: **The Dalai Lama, who believes that "the purpose of life is happiness," also teaches that "happiness can be achieved through training the mind":** His Holiness the Dalai Lama and Howard Cutler, MD, *The Art of Happiness: A Handbook for Living* (New York: Putnam Books, 1998), 13–14: See also: www.1000ventures.com/business_guide/crosscuttings/cultures _buddhism_dalai_lama.html.

67: **Studies show it [MBSR] to be effective at improving outcomes and quality of life in patients with chronic pain and a variety of diseases:** Margaret Plews-Ogan et al., "A Pilot Study Evaluating Mindfulness-Based Stress Reduction and Massage for the Management of Chronic Pain," *Gen Intern Med* 20, no. 12 (December 2005): 1136–38. See also: E. Bohlmeijer et al., "The Effects of Mindfulness-Based Stress Reduction Therapy on Mental Health of Adults with a Chronic Medical Disease: A Meta-Analysis," *J Psychosom Res* 68, no. 6 (June 2010): 539–44; and www.mindfullivingprograms.com/whatMBSR.php.

67: **In a study reported in January 2011 in *Psychiatry Research*:** Britta K. Hölzel et al., "Mindfulness Practice Leads to Increases in Regional Brain Gray Matter Density," *Psychiat Res Neuroimaging* 191, no. 1 (January 30, 2011): 36–43.

67: **Another application, mindfulness-based cognitive therapy (MBCT):** www.mindfullivingprograms.com/whatMBSR.php. See also: "Mindfulness-Based Cognitive Therapy," www.mbct .com and Zindel V. Segal et al., "Antidepressant Monotherapy vs. Sequential Pharmacotherapy and Mindfulness-Based Cognitive Therapy, or Placebo, for Relapse Prophylaxis in Recurrent Depression," *Arch Gen Psychiat* 67, no. 12 (December 2010): 1256–64, http://archpsyc.ama-assn.org/cgi/content/short/67/12/1256.

67: **Daniel Siegel, MD, clinical professor of psychiatry at UCLA...calls this ability "mindsight":** Daniel J. Siegel, *Mindsight: The New Science of Personal Transformation* (New York: Bantam Books, 2010), xi–xiii.

CHAPTER 5. Optimizing Emotional Well-Being by Caring for the Body

73: **Up to 20 percent of people suffering from depression are deficient in thyroid hormones:** I. Hickle et al., "Clinical and Subclinical Hypothyroidism in Patients with Chronic and Treatment-Resistant Depression," *Austral NZ J Psychiat* 30 (April 1996): 246–52. See also: "Depression Explored, with Dr. Barry Durrant-Peatfield," November 19, 2003, http://thyroid.about .com/b/2003/11/19/depression-explored-with-dr-barry-durrant -peatfield.htm.

74: **Dysfunction of the pituitary and adrenal glands also commonly affects emotional health, as do the drugs used to treat it:** W. F. Kelly, "Psychiatric Aspects of Cushing's Syndrome," *QJM* 89 (1996): 543–51, http://qjmed.oxfordjournals.org/content/89/7/543 .full.pdf+html?sid=1ce50d74-b3f4-4d2a-b7b0-8d367d3133ee.

74: **Depression in some older men can be relieved by boosting low testosterone levels:** M. Amore et al., "Partial Androgen Deficiency, Depression and Testosterone Treatment in Aging Men," *Aging Clin Exper Res* 21, no. 1 (February 2009): 1–8.

74: **People with diabetes are more likely to be depressed than people without it:** Pan An et al., "Bidirectional Association Between Depression and Type 2 Diabetes Mellitus in Women," *Arch Int Med* 170, no. 21 (November 22, 2010): 1884–91. See also: S. H. Golden et al., "Examining a Bidirectional Association Between Depressive Symptoms and Diabetes," *JAMA* 299, no. 23 (2008): 2751–59.

74: **A recent study in animals with type-1 diabetes demonstrated a previously unknown effect of insulin:** "Insulin's Brain Impact Links Drugs and Diabetes," Vanderbilt University Medical Center, *ScienceDaily*, October 17, 2007, www.sciencedaily.com /releases/2007/10/071017090131.htm.

74 (footnote): **Concern about this possibility in one Addison's sufferer, John F. Kennedy:** Thomas H. Maugh, "John F. Kennedy's

Addison's Disease Was Probably Caused by Rare Autoimmune Disease," *Los Angeles Times,* September 5, 2009, http://articles .latimes.com/print/2009/sep/05/science/sci-jfk-addisons5.

75: **One in three heart attack survivors experiences depression, as does one in four people who have strokes and one in three patients with HIV:** "Co-Occurrence of Depression with Other Illnesses," from National Institute of Mental Health publication "Men and Depression," *NIMH* (2005): www.nimh.nih.gov/health /publications/men-and-depression/co-occurrence-of-depression -with-other-illnesses.shtml.

75: **An even higher percentage—50 percent—of people with Parkinson's disease suffer from depression:** Miranda Hitti, "Depression Common with Parkinson's Disease," *WebMD Health News,* September 29, 2004, www.webmd.com/parkinsons-disease /news/20040929/depression-common-with-parkinsons-disease.

75: **"The depression is part of the illness, not simply a reaction to the disease":** Hitti, "Depression Common."

76: **As many as 25 percent of persons with cancer experience depression:** Dana Jennings, "After Cancer, Ambushed by Depression," *New York Times,* Health Section, September 29, 2009.

76: **With some kinds of cancer—notably pancreatic—the percentage is much higher:** Frank J. Brescia, "Palliative Care in Pancreatic Cancer," *Cancer Control* 11, no. 1 (January/February 2004): 39–45.

77: **A commonly reported side effect of interferon therapy is severe depression; some patients have even killed themselves:** Molly McElroy, "Scientists Build on Case Connecting Inflammatory Disease and Depression," Illinois News Bureau, July 27, 2004, http://news.illinois.edu/news/04/0727depression.html.

77: **In addition to severe physical side effects, it can cause paranoia and hallucinations:** Timothy DiChiara, "What You Need to Know About Interleukin-2 for Metastatic Melanoma"

About.com, March 31, 2009, http://skincancer.about.com/od/treatmentoptions/a/interleukin.htm.

77: **when proinflammatory cytokines are administered to animals, they elicit "sickness behavior":** K. W. Kelley et al., "Cytokine-Induced Sickness Behavior," *Brain Behav Immun* 17, 1 (February, 2003): 112–18.

77: **in the 1960s, research revealed a blood-borne factor to be responsible:** J. E. Holmes and N. E. Miller, "Effects of Bacterial Endotoxin on Water Intake, Food Intake, and Body Temperature in the Albino Rat," *J Exp Med* 118 (1963): 649–58. See also: N. Miller, "Some Psychophysiological Studies of Motivation and of the Behavioral Effects of Illness," *Bull Br Psychol Soc* 17 (1964): 1–20.

80: **These are classified as high-glycemic-load foods because they raise blood sugar quickly:** Jennie Brand-Miller et al., *The Glucose Revolution: The Authoritative Guide to the Glycemic Index* (Emeryville, Calif.: Marlowe & Company, 1999).

81: **People who are fit and who exercise regularly have less inflammation than others:** E. S. Ford, "Does Exercise Reduce Inflammation? Physical Activity and C-reactive Protein Among U.S. Adults," *Epidemiol* 15, no. 5 (September 2002): 561–68: See also: Rainer Rauramaa et al., "Effects of Aerobic Physical Exercise on Inflammation and Atherosclerosis in Men: The DNASCO Study: A Six-Year Randomized, Controlled Trial," *Ann Int Med* 140, no. 12 (June 15, 2004): 1007–14.

81: **The quantity and quality of your sleep also influence inflammation, as does stress:** "Poor Sleep Quality Increases Inflammation, Community Study Finds," *Science Blog*, November 14, 2010, http://scienceblog.com/40178/poor-sleep-quality-increases-inflammation-community-study-finds/. See also: Robert A. Anderson, "Inflammation and Stress," *Townsend Letter for Doctors and Patients,* May 2005, http://findarticles.com/p/articles/mi_m0ISW/is_262/ai_n13675741/; and N. Simpson and

D. F. Dinges, "Sleep and Inflammation," *Nutr Rev* 65, no. 12, part 2, supplement (December 2007): 244–52.

83: **Many studies link specific nutrient deficiencies to subopti-mal brain function and mental/emotional health:** David F. Horrobin, "Food, Micronutrients, and Psychiatry," *Int Psychoge-riat* 14, no. 4 (January, 2005): 331–34.

83: **omega-3 fatty acids. These special fats are critically impor-tant for both physical and mental health:** "Fish Oils and Men-tal Health/Depression," posted on *oilofpisces.com database,* 2010, www.oilofpisces.com/depression.html.

83: **Dietary supplementation with these fats, usually in the form of fish oil, has proved to be an effective, natural, and non-toxic therapy:** "Fish Oils and Mental Health/Depression."

83: **Very high doses of fish oil—20 grams a day or more—have been used as treatments without any ill effects:** "Fish Oils and Mental Health/Depression."

84: **A gorilla, eating mostly leaves and other raw vegetable matter that is very low in fats, has a brain that is about 0.2 percent of overall body weight:** Imonikhe Ahimie, "The Difference Between Human Primates and Ape Primates," posted on *Helium .com,* September 1, 2009, www.helium.com/items/1572554 -differences-between-human-primates-and-ape-primates.

86: **vitamin D, and it is almost impossible to get enough of it from diet alone:** "Vitamin D Important in Brain Development and Function," *Science News,* April 23, 2008, www.sciencedaily .com/releases/2008/04/080421072159.htm.

87: **not just for bone health but for protection against many kinds of cancer, multiple sclerosis, influenza, and other dis-eases:** "Vitamin D Important."

87: **more doctors now routinely check blood levels of vitamin D in their patients and are documenting a deficiency in many of them:** "Vitamin D Important."

87: **High vitamin D levels may protect against age-related cognitive decline:** D. M. Lee et al., "Association Between 25-hydroxyvitamin D Levels and Cognitive Performance in Middle-Aged and Older European Men," *J Neurol Neurosurg Psychiat* 80, no. 7 (Epub May 21, 2009): 722–29.

87: **(The last correlation is posed as a possible explanation for the surprisingly high incidence of schizophrenia in dark-skinned immigrants who move to northern European countries):** M. J. Dealberto, "Why Are Immigrants at Increased Risk for Psychosis? Vitamin D Insufficiency, Epigenetic Mechanisms, or Both?" *Med Hypotheses* 70, no. 1 (2008): 211.

88: **Deficiencies of other vitamins and trace minerals have been reported in people with mood disorders:** David F. Horrobin, "Food, Micronutrients, and Psychiatry," *Int Psychogeriat* 14, no. 4 (January 2005): 331–34.

89: **A national news story from June 2010 described an "unorthodox treatment for anxiety and mood disorders":** Laura Blue, "Is Exercise the Best Drug for Depression?" *Time Magazine Online*, June 19, 2010, www.time.com/time/health/article/0,8599,1998021,00.html.

89: **"In order for man to succeed in life, god provided him with two means":** Plato, 4th century BCE, quoted in Andreas Struohle, "Physical Activity, Exercise, Depression and Anxiety Disorders," *J Neural Transm* 116 (2009): 777–84.

90: **Many studies show that depressed patients who stick to a regimen of aerobic exercise improve as much as those treated with medication and are less likely to relapse:** Struohle, "Physical Activity, Exercise, Depression and Anxiety Disorders."

90: **The data also suggest that exercise prevents depression and boosts mood in healthy people:** Struohle, "Physical Activity, Exercise, Depression and Anxiety Disorders."

90: **Most prospective studies have used walking or jogging programs:** Struohle, "Physical Activity, Exercise, Depression and Anxiety Disorders."

91: **some research finds nonaerobic exercise such as strength and flexibility training as well as yoga to be effective, too:** Struohle, "Physical Activity, Exercise, Depression and Anxiety Disorders." See also: B. G. Bergen and D. R. Owen, "Mood Alteration with Yoga and Swimming: Aerobic Exercise May Not Be Necessary," *Percept Mot Skills* 75, no. 3, part 2 (December 1992): 1331–43.

91: **clinical psychologist and yoga therapist Bo Forbes explains:** Quote following is from Bo Forbes, *Yoga for Emotional Balance*, (Boulder, Colo.: Shambhala Publications, 2010), 39.

91: **The most important conclusions of research to date are that regular physical activity:** Struohle, "Physical Activity, Exercise, Depression and Anxiety Disorders."

95: **Most experts agree that sleep and mood are closely related:** Lawrence J. Epstein, MD, "Sleep and Mood," December 15, 2008, http://healthysleep.med.harvard.edu/need-sleep/whats-in-it-for-you/mood.

95: **Studies report that about 90 percent of patients with major depression have difficulty initiating and maintaining sleep:** Epstein, "Sleep and Mood."

95: **chronic insomnia—on and off for the better part of a year— is a strong clinical predictor of depression:** Epstein, "Sleep and Mood."

95: **Five to 10 percent of the adult population in Western industrialized countries suffer from chronic insomnia:** Epstein, "Sleep and Mood."

95: **Most of it involves sleep deprivation: human subjects are observed in laboratories over days or weeks when they are allowed to sleep less than normal amounts:** Ruth M. Benca, "How Does Sleep Loss Affect Mood?" *Medscape Family Medicine*

7, no. 2 (2005), cme.medscape.com/viewarticle/515564. See also: Monica Haack and Janet M. Mullington, "Sustained Sleep Restriction Reduces Emotional and Physical Well-Being," *Pain* 119, no. 1 (December 15, 2005): 56–64.

95: **One study at the University of Pennsylvania:** David Dinges et al., "Cumulative Sleepiness, Mood Disturbance, and Psychomotor Vigilance Decrements During a Week of Sleep Restricted to 4–5 Hours Per Night," *Sleep* 20, no. 4 (April 1997): 267–77.

96: **Another study, by investigators at Harvard Medical School and the University of California, Berkeley, used functional MRI to assess changes in brain function with sleep deprivation:** Seung-Schik Yoo et al., "The Human Emotional Brain Without Sleep—A Prefrontal Amygdala Disconnect," *Curr Biol* 17, no. 20 (October 23, 2007): R877–78.

96: **because sleep deprivation also increases inflammation in the body:** Deborah Simpson and David F. Dinges, "Sleep and Inflammation," *Nutr Rev* 65 (December 2007): S244–52.

96: **Mood disorders are also strongly linked to…REM (rapid eye movement) sleep:** Rosalind Cartwright, *The Twenty-four Hour Mind: The Role of Sleep and Dreaming in Our Emotional Lives* (New York: Oxford University Press, 2010), 7.

96: **"REM/dream loss is the most critical overlooked sociocultural force in the etiology of depression":** Rubin Naiman, "Circadian Rhythm and Blues: The Interface of Depression with Sleep and Dreams," *Psychology Today Blog by Rubin Naiman, PhD,* February 28, 2011, www.psychologytoday.com/blog/bloggers/rubin-naiman-phd.

96: **Of significance is the fact that most medications used to help people sleep suppress REM sleep and dreaming:** Naiman, "Circadian Rhythm and Blues."

96: **Research suggests that the emotional content of many dreams is negative:** Naiman, "Circadian Rhythm and Blues."

104: **With long-term use, steroids cause emotional instability, mania, and, most often, depression:** S. B. Patten, "Exogenous Corticosteroids and Major Depression in the General Population," *J Psychosom Res* 49, no. 6 (December 2000): 447–49: See also: *Diagnostic and Statistical Manual of Mental Disorders, Fourth Edition, Text Revision* (DSM-IV-TR), published by the American Psychiatric Association, 2000.

105: **(Interestingly, Iceland is an exception, probably because its inhabitants have unusually high tissue levels of omega-3 fatty acids from a diet rich in oily fish, as well as high dietary intake of vitamin D):** Daphne Miller, *The Jungle Effect: Healthiest Diets from Around the World: Why They Work and How to Make Them Work for You* (New York: Harper, 2009), 137–39.

105: **In 1984, Norman E. Rosenthal, MD, and colleagues at the National Institute of Mental Health described a form of depression that recurred seasonally:** N. E. Rosenthal et al., "Seasonal Affective Disorder: A Description of the Syndrome and Preliminary Findings with Light Therapy," *Arch Gen Psychiat* 41, no. 1 (1984): 72–80.

106: **his 1993 book, *Winter Blues,* is the classic treatise on the subject:** Norman E. Rosenthal, *Winter Blues* (New York: Guilford Press, 1993).

106: **An estimated 6.1 percent of the US population suffers from SAD, and more than twice as many people are prone to a milder form called subsyndromal seasonal affective disorder, or SSAD:** D. H. Avery et al., "Bright Light Therapy of Subsyndromal Seasonal Affective Disorder in the Workplace: Morning vs. Afternoon Exposure," *Acta Psychiatrica Scandinavica* 103, no. 4 (2001): 267–74: See also: M. Said, "Seasonal Affective Disorders," *Priory* (January 2001), priory.com/psych/SAD.htm.

106: **Whatever its cause, treatment with full-spectrum light—not the same as ordinary indoor light—works to relieve SAD as**

effectively as antidepressant drugs and faster: Robert N. Golden et al., "The Effect of Light Therapy in the Treatment of Mood Disorders: A Review and Meta-Analysis of the Evidence," *Am J Psychiat* 162 (April 2005): 656–62.

106: **but analysis of data so far suggests that it can be effective for treating nonseasonal depression, again working as well as medication:** Golden, "Effect of Light Therapy."

107: **Many devices include wavelengths of blue light that are hazardous to the eye, increasing the risk of age-related macular degeneration (AMD):** "The Dark Side of Light: Rhodopsin and the Silent Death of Vision. The Proctor Lecture," *Investig Ophthalmol Vis Sci* 46 (2005): 2672–82: See also: "The Risk of Eye Damage from Bright Light and Blue Light Therapy," www.*sunnexbiotech* .*com*, www.sunnexbiotech.com/therapist/main.htm.

107: **(Herbert Kern, the engineer who first tried it, reported in an article in *Science* in 2007):** Y. Bhattacharjee, "Psychiatric Research. Is Internal Timing Key to Mental Health?" *Science* 317, no. 5844 (September 14, 2007): 1488–90.

110: **Long-term use of antidepressant drugs may actually prolong depression:** Rif S. El-Mallakh et al., "Tardive Dysphoria: The Role of Long-term Antidepressant Use in Inducing Chronic Depression," *Med Hypotheses* 76, no. 6 (June 2011): 769–73.

111: **Recent research suggests that antidepressant medications may increase the risk:** Steven Rosenberg, "Study Hints at Link Between Antidepressants and Heart Trouble," report on presentation by Dr. Amit Shah at the 2011 annual meeting of the American College of Cardiology, *HealthDay News,* April 2, 2011; L. Cosgrove, Ling Shi et al., "Antidepressants and Breast and Ovarian Cancer Risk: A Review of the Literature and Researchers' Financial Associations with Industry," *PlosOne,* www.plosone .org/article/info%3Adoi%2F10.1371%2Fjournal.pone.0018210.

112: **This European plant *(Hypericum perforatum)* has a long history of medicinal use, including as an herbal mood booster:**

Paul Hammernes et al., "St. John's Wort: A Systematic Review of Adverse Effects and Drug Interactions for the Consultation Psychiatrist," *Psychosomatics* 44 (August 2003): 271–82.

112: **most experimental results with mild to moderate depression have been positive, with St. John's wort performing better than a placebo, often doing as well as prescription antidepressants, and sometimes proving more effective than the drugs:** Hammernes et al., "St. John's Wort."

114: **SAMe has been extensively studied as an antidepressant and treatment for the pain of osteoarthritis:** "SAMe for Treatment of Depression," *The National Center for Complementary and Alternative Medicine at the National Institutes of Health,* December 22, 2008, www.healthyplace.com/depression/alternative-treatments /same-for-treatment-of-depression/menu-id-68/.

114: **In recent research...investigators from Harvard Medical School and Massachusetts General Hospital gave SAMe or a placebo to seventy-three depressed adults:** George I. Papakostas et al., "S-Adenosyl Methionine (SAMe) Augmentation of Serotonin Reuptake Inhibitors for Antidepressant Nonresponders with Major Depressive Disorder: A Double-Blind, Randomized Clinical Trial," *Am J Psychiat* 167 (August 2010): 942–48.

116: ***Rhodiola rosea:*** Richard P. Brown et al., "*Rhodiola rosea:* A Phytomedicinal Overview," American Botanical Council, *HerbalGram* 56 (2002): 40–52.

116: ***[Rhodiola rosea]* has been extensively studied by scientists in Russia and Sweden:** Brown et al., "*Rhodiola rosea.*"

116: **Rhodiola root contains rosavins, compounds that appear to enhance activity of neurotransmitters in the brain and may be responsible for the herb's beneficial effects on mood and memory:** Brown et al., "*Rhodiola rosea.*"

116: **In a 2007 double-blind, placebo-controlled human study from Sweden:** V. Darbinyan et al., "Clinical Trial of *Rhodiola* *rosea* L. Extract SHR-5 in the Treatment of Mild to Moderate Depression," by *Nordic J Psychiat* 61, no. 5 (2007): 343–48.

117: **Valerian comes from the root of a European plant *(Valeriana officinalis)* used safely for centuries to promote relaxation and sleep:** American Botanical Council, *The ABC Clinical Guide to Herbs* (New York: Thieme Publishers, 2003), 351–64.

117: **Kava is another root with a sedative effect:** *ABC Clinical Guide to Herbs,* 259–71.

117: **Kava is an excellent anti-anxiety remedy, shown in controlled human trials to be as effective as benzodiazepine drugs:** *ABC Clinical Guide to Herbs,* 259–71.

118: **Animal research shows ashwagandha to be equivalent to true Panax ginseng in stress protection, without ginseng's stimulating effect:** "Materia Medica: Withania somnifera," *Europ J Herbal Med* 4, no. 2 (1998): 17–22. See also: S. K. Bhattacharya and A. V. Muruganandam, "Adaptogenic Activity of Withania Somnifera: An Experimental Study Using a Rat Model of Chronic Stress," *Pharmacol Biochem Behav* 75, no. 3 (June 2003): 545–55.

118: **Human studies in India demonstrate ashwagandha's anti-anxiety and mood-elevating properties and confirm its lack of toxicity:** S. K. Kulkarni and A. Dhir, "Withania Somnifera: An Indian Ginseng," *Prog Neuropsychopharmacol Biol Psychiat* 32, no. 5 (July 1, 2008): 1093–1105.

119: **Holy basil, or tulsi *(Ocimum sanctum),* is a sacred plant in India.... Modern research in both animals and humans demonstrates a lack of toxicity and a variety of benefits:** S. Singh et al., "Evaluation of Anti-inflammatory Potential of Fixed Oil of *Ocimum sanctum* (Holy Basil) and Its Possible Mechanism of Action," *J Ethnopharmacol* 54 (1996): 19–26. See also: David Winston and Steven Maimes, *Adaptogens: Herbs for Strength, Stamina, and Stress Relief* (Rochester, Vt.: Inner Traditions—Bear & Co., 2007), and Dr. Narendra Singh and Dr. Yamuna Hoette, *Tulsi—Mother Medicine of Nature,* International Institute of

Herbal Medicine (Lucknow, India), 2002, www.holy-basil
.com/6685.html and www.pharmainfo.net/reviews/ocimum
-sanctum-and-its-therapeutic-applications.

120: **My colleague Jim Nicolai, MD, medical director of the Integrative Wellness Program at Miraval Resort and Spa in Tucson, tells me he has had great success with holy basil in his
patients:** Personal communication, 2010.

121: **Turmeric, the yellow spice that colors curry and American
yellow mustard, is a potent natural anti-inflammatory agent:**
American Botanical Council, *HerbalGram* 84 (2009): 1–3, http://
cms.herbalgram.org/herbalgram/issue84/article3450.html.

121: **Its active constituent, curcumin, has shown promise as an
antidepressant:** S. Kulkarni et al., "Antidepressant Activity of
Curcumin: Involvement of Serotonin and Dopamine System,"
Psychopharmacol 201, no. 3 (September 3, 2008): 435–42.

121: **Indian researchers suggest doing clinical trials to explore its
efficacy as a novel antidepressant:** S. Kulkarni et al., "Potentials
of Curcumin as an Antidepressant," *Scientific World J* 9 (November 2009): 1233–41.

121: **absorption is greatly increased by the presence of piperine, a
compound in black pepper:** G. Shoba et al., "Influence of
Piperine on the Pharmacokinetics of Curcumin in Animals
and Human Volunteers," *Planta Med* 64, no. 4 (May 1998):
353–56.

121: **in a controlled trial from China in 1994, depressed patients
treated six times a week with acupuncture for six weeks
improved as much as those treated with amitriptylene (Elavil):**
X. Yang et al., "Clinical Observation on Needling Extrachannel
Points in Treating Mental Depression," *J Tradit Chin Med* 14, no.
1 (March 1994): 14–18. See also: Pavel Jalynytchev and Valen-
tina Jalynytchev, "Role of Acupuncture in the Treatment of
Depression, Benefits and Limitations of Adjunctive Treatment
and Monotherapy," *Psychiat Times* 26, no. 6 (May 12, 2009),

www.psychiatrictimes.com/depression/content/article
/10168/1413274.

122: **Some studies use electroacupuncture:** G. A. Ulett et al., "Electroacupuncture: Mechanisms and Clinical Application," *Biol Psychiat* 44, no. 2 (July 15, 1998): 129–38.

122: **We know that animal and human infants deprived of physical contact do not develop normally; some actually sicken and die:** Katherine Harmon, "How Important Is Physical Contact with Your Infant?" *Scientific American Newsletters* (May 6, 2010): www.scientificamerican.com/article.cfm?id=infant-touch.

122: **Some new, intriguing studies are documenting the biochemical benefits of touch:** Mark Hyman Rapaport et al., "A Preliminary Study of the Effects of a Single Session of Swedish Massage on Hypothalamic-Pituitary-Adrenal and Immune Function in Normal Individuals," *J Compl Alt Med* 16, no. 10 (October 18, 2010): 1079–88.

123: **Touch promotes the release of oxytocin, which in turn causes the release of dopamine in the brain's reward center:** Paul J. Zak et al., "The Neurobiology of Trust," *Ann New York Acad Sci* 1032 (2004): 224–27.

123: **Paul J. Zak, PhD, a founder of the contemporary field of neuroeconomics:** Paul Zak with Susan Kuchinskas, "The Power of a Handshake: How Touch Sustains Personal and Business Relationships," *Huffington Post,* September 29, 2008, www.huffingtonpost.com/paul-j-zak/the-power-of-a-handshake_b_129441.html.

124: **The brains of those who got massage released more oxytocin than the brains of those who rested. And the massaged subjects returned 243 percent more money to the strangers who showed them trust:** Vera B. Morhenn et al., "Monetary Sacrifice Among Strangers Is Mediated by Endogenous Oxytocin Release After Physical Contact," *Evol Human Behav* 29, no. 6 (November 2008): 375–83.

124: **An article with the provocative title "Is Dirt the New Prozac?":** Josie Glausiusz, *Discover,* July 2007, http://discovermagazine.com/2007/jul/raw-data-is-dirt-the-new-prozac.

CHAPTER 6. Optimizing Emotional Well-Being by Retraining and Caring for the Mind

129: **Mark Twain advised to "drag your thoughts away from your troubles...by the ears, by the heels, or any other way you can manage it":** Popularly attributed to Mark Twain.

130: **the field known as positive psychology is quite recent. Its chief proponent is Martin Seligman:** Martin E. P. Seligman, *Authentic Happiness: Using the New Positive Psychology to Realize Your Potential for Lasting Fulfillment* (New York: Free Press, 2004).

130: **"Remember that foul words or blows in themselves are no outrage, but your judgment that they are so":** Quote attributed to Epictetus (55–135 CE), *Internet Encyclopedia of Philosophy,* 2011, www.iep.utm.edu/epictetu.

132: **Seligman has tested many interventions to help people enjoy greater pleasure, flow, and meaning in their lives and has found three to be particularly effective:** Seligman, *Authentic Happiness.*

135: **American psychiatrist Aaron T. Beck (1921–), who developed a cognitive theory of depression in the 1960s, is regarded as the father of cognitive therapy:** http://en.wikipedia.org/wiki/Aaron_Temkin_Beck.

135: **(In his original treatment manual, Beck wrote, "The philosophical origins of cognitive therapy can be traced back to the Stoic philosophers"):** A. T. Beck et al., *Cognitive Therapy of Depression* (New York: Guilford Press, 1979), 8.

136: **In a 2011 publication, the British Royal College of Psychiatrists concluded that CBT:** Bullet points following are from "Cognitive Behavioural Therapy (CBT)," *Royal College of*

Psychiatrists, 2011, http://rcpsych.ac.uk/mentalhealthinformation /therapies/cognitivebehaviouraltherapy.aspx?theme.

136: **Depressive symptoms often improve in this initial stage, and many patients are no longer depressed after only eight to twelve sessions:** A. C. Butler and A. T. Beck, "Cognitive Therapy for Depression," *The Clinical Psychologist* 48, no. 3 (1995): 3–5.

137: **In a study reported in the December 2010 issue of the *Archives of General Psychiatry:*** Zindel V. Segal et al., "Antidepressant Monotherapy vs. Sequential Pharmacotherapy and Mindfulness-Based Cognitive Therapy, or Placebo, for Relapse Prophylaxis in Recurrent Depression," *Arch Gen Psychiat* 67, no. 12 (December 2010): 1256–64.

142: **"The elephant steps right along with his stick held upright in a steady trunk":** Eknath Easwaran, *Meditation: A Simple Eight-Point Program for Translating Spiritual Ideals into Daily Life,* (Tomales, Calif.: Nilgiri Press, 1991), 58.

142: **Using Easwaran's *The Mantram Handbook*, several researchers have documented the efficacy of this method:** Eknath Easwaran, *The Mantram Handbook: A Practical Guide to Choosing Your Mantram and Calming Your Mind,* (Tomales, Calif.: Nilgiri Press, 2008).

142: **One study, published in the *Journal of Continuing Education in Nursing* in 2006:** Jill E. Bormann et al., "Relationship of Frequent Mantram Repetition to Emotional and Spiritual Well-Being in Healthcare Workers," *J Cont Educ Nursing* 37, no. 5 (September/October 2006): 218–24.

143: **Other researchers have come to similar conclusions after testing mantram repetition in male veterans and HIV-positive individuals:** Jill E. Bormann and Adam W. Carrico, "Increases in Positive Reappraisal Coping During a Group-Based Mantram Intervention Mediate Sustained Reductions in Anger in HIV-Positive Persons," *Int J Behav Med* 16, no. 1 (January 2009): 74–80. See also: J. E. Bormann et al., "Mantram Repetition for Stress

Management in Veterans and Employees: A Critical Incident Study," *J Adv Nurs* 53, no. 5 (March 2006): 502–12.

144: **(C. J. Jung incorporated the use of mandala into his psychoanalytic work with patients):** Gerald Schueler, "Chaos Theory: Interface with Jungian Psychology," 1997, www.schuelers.com/chaos/chaos1.htm.

148: **"A Wandering Mind Is an Unhappy Mind" is the title of a report:** Matthew A. Killingsworth and Daniel T. Gilbert, *Science* 300, no. 6006 (November 12, 2010): 932.

150: **"If you can recognize, even occasionally, the thoughts that go through your mind as simply thoughts":** Quote from Eckhart Tolle, *Stillness Speaks* (Vancouver, B.C.: Namaste Publishing, 2003), 14–15.

150: **I wrote about the value of meditation in my first book, *The Natural Mind,* back in 1972:** Andrew Weil, *The Natural Mind* (Boston: Houghton Mifflin Company, 1972).

152: **In his compelling recent book, *In Pursuit of Silence: Listening for Meaning in a World of Noise,* essayist George Prochnik tells a story of going on patrol with a Washington, DC, police officer named John Spencer:** Excerpt that follows is from George Prochnik, *In Pursuit of Silence: Listening for Meaning in a World of Noise* (New York: Doubleday, 2010), 17–18.

156: **"We get much more information than we desire":** Excerpt is from Francis Heylighen, "Complexity and Information Overload in Society: Why Increasing Efficiency Leads to Decreasing Control," Free University of Brussels, 2002 (draft for *The Information Society*), http://pespmc1.vub.ac.be//Papers/Info-Overload.pdf.

162: **In 1900, only 5 percent of US households were single-person households:** "Loneliness and Isolation: Modern Health Risks," *The Pfizer Journal* 4, no. 4 (2000).

163: **A 2006 study in the *American Sociological Review* found that Americans on average had only two close friends to confide**

in, down from an average of three in 1985: Miller McPherson et al., "Social Isolation in America: Changes in Core Discussion Networks Over Two Decades," *Am Soc Rev* 71, no. 3 (2006): 353–75.

163: **Social isolation and loneliness are strongly correlated with depression:** R. A. Schoevers et al., "Risk Factors for Depression in Later Life; Results of a Prospective Community Based Study (AMSTEL)," *J Affect Disord* 59, no. 2 (August 2000): 127–37.

163: **In his classic work,** *Suicide,* **Émile Durkheim (1858–1917), the father of modern sociology, wrote:** Émile Durkheim, *Suicide* (New York: Free Press, 1997), 210.

163: **Researchers have documented an association between Internet use and social isolation as well as depression among adolescents:** Carole Hughes, "The Relationship of Use of the Internet and Loneliness Among College Students," Boston College Dissertations and Theses, Paper AAI9923427, January 1, 1999, http://escholarship.bc.edu/dissertations/AAI9923427/. See also: Kimberly S. Young and Robert C. Rodgers, "The Relationship Between Depression and Internet Addiction," *Cyber Psychol Behav* 1, no. 1 (1998): 25–28; Christopher E. Sanders et al., "The Relationship of Internet Use to Depression and Social Isolation Among Adolescents," *Health Publications*, summer 2000, http://findarticles.com/p/articles/mi_m2248/is_138_35/ai_66171001/pg_2/.

CHAPTER 7. Secular Spirituality and Emotional Well-Being

170: **Mind/body medicine is coming into its own, and more scientists are taking placebo responses seriously:** Harald Walach and Wayne B. Jonas, "Placebo Research: The Evidence Base for Harnessing Self-Healing Capacities," *J Alt Comp Med* 10, no. 1 (2004): S103–12.

173: **A great deal of scientific research confirms the benefits to health in general and emotional health in particular of living with**

companion animals: J. Nimer and B. Lundahl, "Animal Assisted Therapy: A Meta-Analysis," *Anthrozoo* 20, no. 3 (2007): 225–38.

170: **Lynette A. Hart, PhD, a professor of veterinary medicine at the University of California, Davis, writes:** Lynette A. Hart, "Companion Animals Enhancing Human Health and Wellbeing (Proceedings)," *CVC Proceedings,* August 1, 2008, http://veterinarycalendar.dvm360.com/avhc/content/printContentPopup.jsp?id=567242.

170: **"Being around pets appears to feed the soul, promoting a sense of emotional connectedness and overall well-being":** Dennis Thompson Jr., "Pet Therapy and Depression," *Everyday Health,* 2011, www.everydayhealth.com/depression/pet-therapy-and-depression.aspx.

174: **"It is important to develop and uplift human consciousness through beauty," he wrote:** Quote attributed to Mokichi Okada (1882–1955), http://ikebanasangetsu.org/.

176: **In his 2001 book, *The Healing Power of Doing Good:*** Allan Luks, *The Healing Power of Doing Good* (New York: Fawcett Columbine, 1991).

176: **lawyer Allan Luks introduced the term "helper's high" to describe the rush of good feelings that people get when they help others:** Luks, *Healing Power of Doing Good,* xiii.

176: **Since then, neuroscientists have demonstrated that helping others activates the same centers in the brain involved in dopamine-mediated pleasure responses to food and sex:** Shoshana Alexander and James Baraz, "The Helper's High," *The Greater Good,* February 1, 2010, http://greatergood.berkeley.edu/article/item/the_helpers_high/.

176: **In one study, these pleasure centers lit up when participants simply thought about giving money to a charity:** Alexander and Baraz, "Helper's High."

176: **From a study of more than three thousand volunteers, Luks concluded that regular helpers are ten times more likely to be** in good health than people who don't volunteer: Luks, *Healing Power of Doing Good*, xi.

176: **"giving help to others protects overall health twice as much as aspirin protects against heart disease":** Quote and excerpt following are from Christine L. Carter, "What We Get When We Give," *Psychology Today*, February 18, 2010, www.psychologytoday.com.

177: **One of the findings of the landmark Social Capital Community Benchmark Survey of almost thirty thousand Americans, published in 2000:** A. C. Brooks, "Does Giving Make Us Prosperous?" *J Econ Finance* 31, no. 3 (fall 2007): 403–11.

177: **Is charity "really self-interest masquerading under the form of altruism":** Anthony de Mello, *Awareness: A De Mello Spirituality Conference in His Own Words*, edited by J. Francis Stroud (New York: Random House, 1992), 19.

177: **The Dalai Lama uses the term *selfish altruism* without any pejorative sense:** Alexander and Baraz, "Helper's High."

179: **"compassion and affection help the brain to function more smoothly":** Quote is from the Dalai Lama, "Compassion Is the Source of Happiness," *The Berzin Archives*, May 2008, www.berzinarchives.com/web/en/archives/sutra/level2_lamrim/advanced_scope/bodhichitta/compassion_source_happiness.html.

180: **In his brain-imaging studies, Richard Davidson and colleagues have documented changes in the brains of both Tibetan monks and laypersons trained in compassion meditation:** Antoine Lutz et al., "Regulation of the Neural Circuitry of Emotion by Compassion Meditation: Effects of Meditative Expertise," *PLoS ONE* 3, no. 3 (2008).

180: **In his excellent book *The Compassionate Mind*, psychologist Paul Gilbert:** Quotes that follow are from Paul Gilbert, *The Compassionate Mind* (London: Constable, 2009).

181: **"always forgive your enemies—nothing annoys them so much":** Quote popularly attributed to Oscar Wilde.

181: **Research shows that those who forgive enjoy better social interactions in general and become more altruistic over time:** C. V. Witvliet et al., "Forgiveness and Health: Review and Reflections on a Matter of Faith, Feelings, and Physiology," *J Psychol Theol* 29 (2001): 212–24. See also: C. V. Witvliet and K. A. Phipps, "Granting Forgiveness or Harboring Grudges: Implications for Emotion, Physiology, and Health," *Psychol Sci* 12 (2001): 117–23.

181: **a 2009 study documents an inverse correlation between forgiveness and depression:** J. L. Burnette et al., "Insecure Attachment and Depressive Symptoms: The Mediating Role of Rumination, Empathy, and Forgiveness," *Personality and Individual Differences* 46, no. 3 (February 2009): 276–80.

182: **such as a six-hour "empathy-oriented forgiveness seminar":** Stephen J. Sandage and Everett L. Worthington, "Comparison of Two Group Interventions to Promote Forgiveness: Empathy as a Mediator of Change," *J Mental Health Couns* 32, no. 1 (January, 2010): 35–57.

182: **"For me it was a limitation that we were so bound from connecting the material, tangible, and measurable world to spiritual questions and pursuits":** Quote is from Frederic Luskin, MD, in Teresa Rose, "Director of the Stanford Forgiveness Project Frederic Luskin Suggests Forgiving to Mediators" (video), *Examiner.com,* San Francisco, June 4, 2010, www.examiner.com/sf-in -san-francisco/director-of-the-stanford-forgiveness-project- frederic-luskin-suggests-forgiving-to-mediators-video.

184: **"the free expression by outward signs of an emotion intensifies it. On the other hand, the repression, as far as this is possible, of all outward signs softens our emotions....Even the simulation of an emotion tends to arouse it in our minds":** Quote is attributed to Charles Darwin in his *Expression of the Emotions in Man and Animals* (London: John Murray, 1872). See also: Charles Darwin, *The Expression of the Emotions in Man and*

Animals, Joe Cain and Sharon Messenger, eds. (New York: Penguin, 2009), xxviii.

184: **A 1988 study by researchers at Universität Mannheim, Federal Republic of Germany, did just that:** F. Stack et al., "Inhibiting and Facilitating Conditions of the Human Smile: A Nonobtrusive Test of the Facial Feedback Hypothesis," *J Pers Soc Psychol* 54, no. 5 (May 1988): 768-77.

185: **similar studies demonstrate clearly that emotions stimulate physical expressions, *and* physical expressions stimulate emotions:** Studies include: M. Zuckerman et al., "Facial, Autonomic, and Subjective Components of Emotion: the Facial Feedback Hypothesis Versus Externalizer-Internalizer Distinction," *J Pers Soc Psychol* 41 (1981): 929–44; R. Tourangeau and P. C. Ellsworth, "The Role of Facial Response in the Experience of Emotion," *J Pers Soc Psychol* 37, no. 9 (September 1979): 1519–31; Pamela K. Adelmann and R. B. Zajonc, "Facial Efference and the Experience of Emotion," *Ann Rev Psychol* 40 (1989): 249–80.

185: **Begun by Dr. Madan Kataria, a physician from Mumbai, India, the first laughter club convened in March of 1995 with a handful of people:** "What Is Laughter Yoga?" www.laughteryoga.org/index.php?option=com_content&view=article&id=180:what-is-laughter-yoga&catid=85:about-laughter-yoga&Itemid=265.

186: **regular participation in laughter clubs has been shown to improve long-term emotional and physical health in a variety of ways:** "Laughter Lowers Blood Pressure," July 21, 2008, www.laughteryoga.org/index.php?option=com_content&view=category&id=125&layout=blog&Itemid=275&limitstart=160.

187: **"Why? ...Are we afraid of what we will discover when we come face-to-face with ourselves there?":** Quote from Susan Hill, "Silence, Please," *StandPoint Magazine*, June 2009. www.standpointmag.co.uk/silence-please-features-june-09-susan-hill.

187: **"silence is a rich and fertile soil in which many things grow and flourish":** Hill, "Silence, Please."

188: **We now have scientific evidence for emotional contagion:** Alison L. Hill, et al., "Emotions as Infectious Diseases in a Large Social Network: the SISa Model," *Proc Biol Sci* 277, no. 1701 (December 22, 2010): 3827–35.

188: **if you have a happy friend who lives within a mile of you, your chance of happiness increases by 25 percent:** James H. Fowler and Nicholas A. Christakis, "Dynamic Spread of Happiness in a Large Social Network: Longitudinal Analysis over 20 Years in the Framingham Heart Study," *BMJ* 337, no. a2338 (December 4, 2008).

188: **That is one finding of a study published in the *British Medical Journal* in 2008:** Fowler and Christakis, "Dynamic Spread of Happiness."

189: **Other analyses of the same data show that negative emotions are just as transmissible as positive ones.... The same is true of depression:** Michael Yapko, *Depression Is Contagious: How the Most Common Mood Disorder Is Spreading Around the World and How to Stop It* (New York: Free Press, 2009).

189: **We have strong evidence of the power of gratitude to boost mood:** Discussion that follows is from research by Robert Emmons. See: Robert A. Emmons, *Thanks! How Practicing Gratitude Can Make You Happier* (New York: Houghton Mifflin Harcourt, 2007).

190: **regularly practicing grateful thinking can move your emotional set point for happiness by as much as 25 percent in the right direction:** Brad Lemley, "Shiny Happy People: Can You Reach Nirvana with the Aid of Science?" *Discover,* August 2006, http://discovermagazine.com/2006/aug/shinyhappy.

191: **"First, gratitude is acknowledgment of goodness in one's own life":** Emmons, *Thanks!,* 4

192: **The method used most frequently in research on the effects of practicing gratitude is the Gratitude Journal:** Alvaro Fernandez, "Enhance Happiness and Health by Cultivating Gratitude: Interview with Robert Emmons," *SharpBrains*, November 29, 2007, www.sharpbrains.com/blog/2007/11/29/robert-emmons-on-the-positive-psychology-of-gratitude/.

193: **"The thankful receiver bears a plentiful harvest":** *The Complete Poetry & Prose of William Blake,* edited by David V. Erdman et al. (New York: Anchor; rev. ed., 1997), 37.

Index

About the Author

Andrew Weil, MD, is a world-renowned leader and pioneer in the field of integrative medicine, a healing-oriented approach to health care that encompasses body, mind, and spirit.

Dr. Weil is the founder and director of the Arizona Center for integrative Medicine at the University of Arizona Health Sciences Center, where he is also a clinical professor of medicine, professor of public health, and the Lovell-Jones Professor of Integrative Rheumatology. Dr. Weil received both his medical degree and his undergraduate degree in biology (botany) from Harvard University.

Dr. Weil is an internationally recognized expert on maintaining a healthy lifestyle, healthy aging, and the future of medicine and health care. Approximately 10 million copies of Dr. Weil's books have been sold, including *True Food*, *Spontaneous Healing*, *8 Weeks to Optimum Health*, *Eating Well for Optimum Health*, *The Healthy Kitchen*, and *Healthy Aging*.

He is the editorial director of www.drweil.com, the leading Web resource for healthy living based on the philosophy of integrative medicine. He authors the popular "Self-Healing" special publications and is the director of Integrative Health and Healing at Miraval Resort in Tucson, Arizona. As a columnist for *Prevention* magazine and frequent guest on numerous national shows, Dr. Weil provides valuable insight and information on how to make best use of both conventional and complementary medicine in order to optimize the body's natural healing power.